Patient Care Evaluation in Mental Health Programs

Contributors
Lee D. Brauer
M. Harvey Brenner
Solomon Cytrynbaum
Phillip B. Goldblatt
Jerzy E. Henisz
Jerome K. Myers
Eugene S. Paykel
Donald C. Riedel
Carol Schwartz
Gary L. Tischler
Myrna M. Weissman

Patient Care Evaluation in Mental Health Programs

edited by
Donald C. Riedel
Gary L. Tischler
Jerome K. Myers

Ballinger Publishing Company ● Cambridge, Mass.
A Subsidiary of J.B. Lippincott Company

International Standard Book Number: 0-88410-118-5

Library of Congress Catalog Card Number: 74-17414

Printed in the United States of America

Library of Congress Cataloging in Publication Data
Main entry under title:

Patient care evaluation in mental health programs.
   Includes bibliographical references.
   1. Mental health services—Evaluation. 2. Community mental health services—Evaluation. I. Riedel, Donald C., 1934-   ed. II. Tischler, Gary L., ed.
III. Myers, Jerome Keeley, ed. [DNLM: 1. Community mental health services.
2. Patient care planning. WM30 R551p 1974]
RA790.5.P37   362.2'2   74-17414
ISBN 0-88410-118-5

Contents

List of Figures

List of Tables

Foreword

This book identifies and describes mechanisms for patient care evaluation in mental health center programs. Evaluation has become an extra-ordinarily popular word in the health and mental health fields over the past few years. Funders demand it, new structures are being established to do it, and arguments mount about the relevance of peer, expert and consumer review. Happily, some individuals have long been actively engaged in thinking about, establishing and testing patient care evaluation structures and processes in mental health centers.

Much of the work which led to this book was conducted at the Connecticut Mental Health Center. Dr. Gerald Klerman, Director of the Center from August 1967 to September 1969, helped to stimulate the interest of psychiatrists in the process of utilization review and patient care evaluation. During this same period, the Department of Mental Health in the State of Connecticut was actively engaged in examining data systems for use within state facilities. Dr. Klerman's influence in promoting evaluative studies and the state's interest in upgrading data systems for the department of mental health led the center to become affiliated with the Multi-State Information System in July 1969. Shortly thereafter the Center was selected as a site for the Psychiatric Utilization Review and Evaluation Project. This volume presents the results of the Project's work in establishing an evaluative structure and provides the reader a model for a systematic and cohesive approach to patient care evaluation in mental health settings.

The work of patient care evaluation is complex and, in its formative stages, demands the skills of members of many disciplinary groups. In this volume, authors representing the disciplines of sociology, psychiatry, epidemiology and public health, psychology and social work document their collaboration. They (chapter 1) identify a number of illness perspectives which influence treatment orientations, and which are acknowledged to be more or less valuable in regard to planning care for differing psychiatric conditions. They adopt an eclectic position in regard to patient care evaluation which draws upon four perspectives about psychiatric disorders: (1) psychological-developmental, (2) ecologic, (3) biologic and (4) learning.

Evaluation begins with an examination of what is—and the editors of this book correctly point out that it is—therefore, relative and judgemental, reflecting present knowledge and opinion and dominant values. Most of the work represented in the book stresses ecologic and biologic perspectives although the framework can encompass evaluative efforts directed towards conditions and treatment efforts which may lie predominantly in the psychological-developmental area and in the learning area.

The framework for evaluation also considers treatment and institutional phenomena which interact with ways of looking at individual distress. The focus on the institution stresses examination of *structure* (including the influence of catchmenting (chapter 4) and the utilization of data systems (chapter 3); *processes,* including the development of criteria and their testing and implementation (chapters 5 and 6); and *outcome* (chapter 9).

In their analysis of structural influences, (chapter 1) the authors focus on organizational aspects which influence patient care including personnel, equipment, information and records systems, formal organizational characteristics and financing. They identify the formal role characteristics of staff which may influence care (professional training, role relationships, time commitments and organizational hierarchies). They do not comment upon the personal characteristics of role occupants which may be of importance in psychotherapeutic work in those areas in which the conceptual model of distress is psychological-developmental.

The careful delineation of major psychiatric tasks can allow for the examination of structure, process and outcome in an integrated manner. My colleagues (D.J. Levinson and D. Adler) and I have identified four socially sanctioned major task areas in psychiatry. These include: (1) medical, healing and caring, (2) control of deviancy, (3) habilitative and rehabilitative and (4) existential and humanistic task areas. It is not clear to us that all these tasks can be accomplished in the same organization. They certainly require different work structures and role relationships; they have distinct values associated with task performance, discrete treatment processes and differing preferred outcomes. However, we do not now know of any psychiatric organizations that are structured to address tasks as we have defined them. The authors' charge to develop a mechanism for psychiatric patient care evaluation could not await new structures. Evaluation addresses that which is! Through their careful examination of current practice and through the development and testing of criteria, the authors established a structure and process for patient care evaluation. Their work serves as a vehicle for peer groups to monitor the quality and appropriateness of care, and it also identifies appropriate input for consumers into the evaluative process (chapter 11).

They identify the manner in which individual patient care evaluation serves to monitor the quality of treatment and care within the institution. Data accumulated from many individuals are analyzed to provide information about patterns of care and programmatic and organizational functioning.

Underlying much of the work of this book is an inherent social systems theoretical perspective. The community mental health center is an open system with discrete *input, throughput* and *output* subsystems. An open system is continually engaged in transacting with its environment. It receives inputs from the environment, transforms its inputs and, in order to survive, exports a more valued product to the environment.

Drawing upon experience and research in the field of organizational behavior, the community mental health center is examined in order to identify those points in the organization where major decisions are made about patient care (e.g. entry into the system, transfer between units, discharge) and to investigate the influence of structure and process on care. The assumption is made that separate organizational functions may be profitably examined; that the evaluation of movement into and out of the community mental health center and into and through treatment modalities will provide insights into the nature and quality of the patient care activities of the organization.

In the past decade, particular attention has been paid to issues of admission into treatment systems and to the design of *input structures.* Questions of equal accessibility have been explored. Who is served by the center? Are the poor excluded? Do members of minority groups apply for services? Do they enter into all center programs equally? Is admission into treatment related to severity of pathology, etc.?

In this volume, a number of ways of examining the entry population are presented (chapter 4). Henisz et al. properly stress that a major value of community mental health centers must be to assure equal accessibility to all regardless of race, social class, age, etc. The entry population's demography is described and compared to the population at large. The reasons for seeking out services are identified. Comparisons of populations served to populations within a service area may help to indicate new programmatic directions. Establishing methods for assessing the severity of symptomatology, the availability of social supports and the seriousness of suicidal attempts, etc., may help to insure that applicants for service are adequately evaluated and appropriately treated.

Addressing the issues of input into a system has major implications for design of *throughput structures.* Treatment subsystems must be available to meet patient needs (as identified in the admission process). Tischler (chapter 5) identifies methods of examining appropriateness of treatment modality. Treatment interventions may be characterized by their intensity, goals and structure.

Treatment intensity may encompass a range of services from seeing a patient on an outpatient basis fifteen minutes once a month to weekly or even daily outpatient visits, to day hospital treatment for eight hours a day for five days a week, to inpatient treatment, twenty-four hours a day, seven days a week. Generally, more intense services imply greater patient pathology or need for structure although psychoanalytic psychotherapy (particularly on a multiple visit per week basis) and supportive treatment for chronic patients (on a bimonthly or monthly basis) are exceptions. The goals of treatment may range from crisis intervention, to supportive treatment, to symptomatic modification, to the modification of interpersonal relationships, to uncovering psychotherapy, etc.

Treatment may be structured in individual, group, family or milieu treatment settings with services delivered by diverse professionals or paraprofessionals. Authority relationships may be structured in qualitatively different ways. The therapist may behave as expert, prescribing care to a passively accepting patient. The therapist as expert may attempt to negotiate with the patient to have the patient participate actively and meaningfully in his own therapy. The therapist may act as a participant in the treatment process helping the patient define his own needs, working with the patient so that the patient learns to assume a status similar to that of therapist.

Standards for assignment to treatment can be based upon scientifically established guidelines, current practice, theoretical assumptions, consumer demand, societal insistence or some mix of any or all of these. In this area, there are few studies which clearly document advantages in selecting one or another focus or structure for treatment although clinicians assume that their judgments are reasonable. In chapter 5, some indications for assignment to treatment are explored. Intensity of treatment, particularly the decision to hospitalize, is more frequently related to demonstrable standards (most often, severity of symptomatology). Weissman (chapter 8) elegantly demonstrates in regard to suicidal behavior how decisions as to hospitalization can be carefully examined and criteria refined so that they may guide practice.

Standards for admission to treatment allow decision-making to be examined and standards to be revised in the light of evidence. Obviously far more research is required before evaluative techniques can do more than just maintain current standards of practice.

Once the patient is assigned to some treatment status, the processes of treatment may then be investigated to insure conformity with institutional practice and to review deviant practice as part of an institution's educational responsibility. A number of chapters in this volume (6, 7 and 11) identify approaches to performing case review within institutional settings and have direct applicability to those engaged in setting up evaluative systems in mental health centers. This material and the chapter on data needs for patient care evaluation will probably be of greatest practical utility to those engaged in utilization review and patient care evaluation in mental health facilities. The papers describe the processes involved in developing systems for evaluation, they document the approaches utilized and point to ways in which others may develop systems for individual facility needs. They then detail the procedures of evaluation so that others may rapidly implement them.

Possibly because so much of psychiatric practice is concerned with problems of chronicity, the conceptualization and development of *output structures* is far less evident in psychiatric institutions. Although little attention has been paid to output structures, outcome of care is at times studied as one tool in patient care evaluation. Patients can leave treatment systems even when those systems have no identified output structures. In this area, examination of outcome does not shed light on output structures (in distinction to the input and throughput areas). Most commonly, outcome is examined by exploring patient status at discharge or at some time after discharge. Schwartz and Myers indicate ways in which symptomatic state, social adjustment and consumer satisfaction can be utilized as outcome measures (chapter 9). At times, referral to other settings is investigated as if this were an outcome function. However, since many referrals should be considered as alternative treatment options, such studies may be more properly included in the arena of the evaluation of assignment to treatment (a throughput function).

Evaluation of outcome is *not* research on the efficacy of treatment and must be carefully identified as a separate function. Evaluation does not proceed from an experimental basis. It examines what is or what has happened for the purpose of informed decision making. It cannot answer larger questions about the ultimate value of various interventions.

Perhaps we might consider the process of evaluation as one type of organizational *output structure*. The evaluative process, including evaluation of outcome, provides new information to the organization which enables it to examine itself and, if necessary, change. By judiciously examining data to determine patterns of utilization by various population groups and by examining the interaction of the institution with client groups and agencies in the environment the organization may identify areas in which service is lacking or is redundant. Thus, evaluation is an *output* function which has influence on the total organization and may lead to changes within it.

Patient care evaluation might be considered to complement health education, community and organizational consultation and perhaps even political efforts which seek to modify the interaction of the organization and its environments. Conceptually, these activities may be considered together. They might be likened to the efforts of a sales section (output function) in industry which seeks to interact with and influence its environment in order to get that environment to prize more highly the products of the organization: "We have built a better product, now we must merchandize it." Patient care evaluation, community and organizational consultation, and health education and other indirect services might serve to educate the community, to identify patients as valued members of the community, to focus on their employability, to modify views of mental health and mental illness, to promote health, etc. Seen in this light, evaluation would indeed, be part of an organization's output structure. And then . . . why then, we should of course have to design evaluative studies to determine the efficacy of patient care evaluation.

BORIS M. ASTRACHAN

Acknowledgments

This book is based on the experiences of the Psychiatric Utilization Review and Evaluation (PURE) Project, an interdisciplinary effort conducted as a part of the Health Services Research Program, Institution for Social and Policy Studies, Yale University, by members of several departments of the University and of community mental health centers in four cities, with the cooperation of the Multi-State Information System (MSIS). Funded by the National Institute of Mental Health,[a] it ran more than five years and was dependent upon the dedicated contribution of more than one hundred individuals at various professional levels. We wish to acknowledge here the support of a relatively few of them.

From NIMH: Ruth Knee, Michael Goran, Margaret Conwell, John Burton, Matthew Huxley and Frank Kalibat.

From MSIS: Eugene Laska, Bernice Proctor, Morris Meisner and Mary Jo Ohliger.

From the Erich Lindeman Mental Health Center, Boston: Gerald Klerman (formerly co-principal investigator of PURE while at Yale), Barrett Krasner, James Barrett, Mary Davis, Brooks Mostue and William Huddleston.

From Rockland County Community Mental Health Center, Rockland, New York: Sheldon Zimberg, William Block, Gerald Lee, Marianne Bart and Timothy Moritz.

From Area B Mental Health Center, Washington, D.C.: Jean Tippett, Barbara Smith, Robert Brown, Nancy Tompkins and Eva Rose Towns.

From Connecticut Mental Health Center: The members of the panels and study groups who gave so generously of their time in constructing guidelines for patient care evaluation: Boris Astrachan, Michael Levine, H. Flynn, V. Garrison, J. Henisz, H. Zonana, E. Paykel, D. Dressler, N. French, C. Hallo-

[a]Contract HSM 42–69–60 and Grant USPHS 5–R12–MH–21–354, Donald C. Riedel, Principal Investigator.

well, H. Mark, D. Shapiro, R. Steele, M. Weissman, A. Ward, L. Zegans, J. Geller, J. Schowalter, M. Sullivan, M. Swartzburg, M. Harrow, A. Schwartz, G. Tucker, R. Berberian, B. Prusoff and Oscar Weiner.

Finally, we wish to acknowledge the ongoing assistance provided by Robert Fetter and Ronald Mills, original developers of the interactive computer system known as AUTOGRP which served as the basis for the principal analytic and case selection mechanisms described later.

DONALD C. RIEDEL
GARY L. TISCHLER
JEROME K. MYERS

Patient Care Evaluation in Mental Health Programs

Chapter One

Introduction

Gary L. Tischler
Donald C. Riedel
Jerome K. Myers

Patient care evaluation and utilization review are neither new nor radical concepts. They address themselves to the need for scrutinizing clinical practice in order to maintain the quality of patient care at reasonable levels. The evaluation of patient care includes: (1) comparative study of patients who come to a facility vis-à-vis the total population served; (2) examination of the appropriateness of service allocation and of the priorities assigned to various patients once they are allocated services; (3) analysis of patterns of care; (4) study of service adequacy and quality of care; and (5) the examination of treatment outcome to determine if services are effective. Utilization review is that part of the evaluative endeavor aimed at monitoring the quality of patient care and insuring economical and efficient facility use through an educational approach, involving the study of patterns of care and the encouragement of appropriate utilization.

While segments of the medical profession have long supported evaluative enterprises as viable mechanisms for patient care surveillance, third-party carriers have become increasingly insistent upon their use to insure that program members receive appropriate and economic care. Federally sponsored programs such as Medicare have also begun to include a requirement for patient care evaluation as a condition for participation. Most recently, Professional Standards Review Organizations (PSRO) were established by PL 92–603. The intent of this legislation is to insure effective professional review of the quality and quantity of health care within a context of public accountability.

The emphasis upon assessing health care delivery from both a quantitative and qualitative perspective suggests a shift of focus from issues of cost per se towards considerations related to "getting one's money's worth." This shift is consistent with the more general societal acceptance of the Aristotelian premise that individuals "have an absolute moral right to such a measure of good health as society alone is able to give them," tempered by the emergence of a strong drive towards "consumerism" and catalyzed by the recognition that the health

1

care industry now absorbs over seven percent of the gross national product. A corollary of these events has been the transformation of the delivery, organization, financing and control of health care into a political issue. As a result, there has been not only increased pressure for the more rigorous application of principles of internal accountability, but also growing evidence that self-regulation, as currently practiced by the health care industry, will inevitably give way to more pluralistic systems of public accountability which will include the consumer, third-party agents and the body politic. Within this broader context, patient care evaluation and utilization review may be viewed as potential vehicles for achieving internal accountability through providing more systematic mechanisms for examining and commenting upon propriety of use and quality of care.

THE QUALITY OF PATIENT CARE

Some forty years ago, Lee and Jones [1] propounded eight "articles of faith" defining quality medical care: a scientific basis for medical practice; prevention; accessibility of care for all people; comprehensive and coordinated medical services; treatment of the whole individual; close and continuing patient-physician relations; coordination between medical care and social services; and consumer-provider cooperation. They viewed good medical care as:

> . . . . the kind of medicine practiced and taught by recognized leaders of the medical profession at the given time or period of social, cultural and professional development in the community or population group.

More recently, Payne [2] has described quality care as:

> . . . that level of excellence produced and documented in the process of diagnosis and therapy, based on the best knowledge derived from science and the humanities, and which eventuates in the least morbidity and mortality in the population.

Within the mental health field, Zusman and Lawson [3] have articulated a set of basic assumptions underlying any assessment of the quality of patient care:

1. Good care is recognizable and worth striving for.
2. Decisions regarding the appropriateness of particular mental health services or treatments are embedded within decision makers' value systems and these judgments are subjective.
3. Experts can agree generally on standards of good care.
4. Elements of good care can be characterized and rated.
5. The definition of "good" depends upon present knowledge and opinion.

Taken together, these statements portray patient care as a process strongly influenced by those conceptual models operant within a field at a particular point in time. It follows, therefore, that a definition of good care will be both relative—in that it reflects present knowledge and opinion—and judgmental —in that, where more than one conceptual model exists, good will be phrased in terms of the dominant value system. This, in turn, complicates the assessment of quality, since the evaluative process must contend with the level of confirmation achieved by the constructs forming the conceptual base upon which patient care activities rest. While the evaluative process need not accept these constructs as facts, it should attend to their very real influence upon the nature of patient care and their use as benchmarks against which practitioners measure the success or failure of particular treatment interventions. Similarly, knowledge of the various constructs operant within a particular field also enhances the evaluator's understanding of clinical practice and provides the basis for a more explicit dialogue with the practitioner.

ILLNESS PERSPECTIVES AND TREATMENT ORIENTATIONS

Within the mental health field, it is possible to identify four illness perspectives that exert a major influence upon contemporary clinical practice: the psycho-social-developmental perspective; the ecologic perspective; the biologic perspective; and the learning perspective. Each perspective attempts to explain the origin and nature of disordered behavior. These explanations, in turn, influence the evolution of particular treatment orientations.

The Psychosocial-Developmental Perspective

According to this perspective, mental disorder develops as the result of some specific deprivation or interference that occurs during a critical period of psychological development. Disordered and normal behavior are viewed as falling on a continuum and explained on the basis of theories governing our understanding of normal personality development. While traditional psychodynamic views have been modified, to account for the complex outcomes of interactions between the individual personality and the social environment, emphasis is still placed upon the importance of intrapsychic factors. As a result, a strong bias exists that the source of difficulty lies within an individual and can be alleviated or remedied through changing some aspect of personality.

Therapy makes use of verbal and symbolic techniques aimed at producing personality change. While constantly striving to create a working alliance with the patient, the therapist consistently maintains the position that growth, maturation and change will come as the patient works towards greater self-understanding. Some therapists feel that this self-understanding stems from the emergence of new insights that result from a clarification of the psychological meaning of events, feelings and behaviors. Others see it as a derivative of the patient-therapist relationship—a relationship that fosters the remembrance of highly charged experiences, facilitates working these experiences through, and encourages the patient to move beyond them and abandon pathologic ways of coping.

The Ecologic Perspective

The ecologic perspective focuses upon aspects of the relationship between man and his environment. The broad parameters of acceptable and unacceptable behavior reflect the norms operative within a particular society or culture at a given time. An individual who deviates from these norms is regarded as potentially or actually ill. While there are predictable patterns of individual behavior characteristic of any one social situation, the expressive behavior of individuals changes in newly defined social settings. Given sufficient deprivation or stress producing stimuli or other alterations in the environment, behavior can be altered to a point where the ability to cope or adapt is severely compromised. Mentally ill behavior is thus judged in relation to the context in which it unfolds.

Treatment interventions focus less upon growth and maturation than upon adaptation, coping and integration with the environment. Where social stress is so severe that it taxes coping ability and causes severe disability, approaches that alleviate stress or enhance coping are used. These involve instruction, support and encouragement. The therapist may also work to reestablish the social field within which the patient functions. This can involve a direct intervention as an advocate, expediter or facilitator or efforts at restructuring a nuclear social system through the use of family therapy. Additionally, the ecologic perspective encourages clinicians to view treatment modalities as transitional social systems, with resultant emphasis upon the use and validity of milieu and group therapy techniques.

The Biologic Perspective

This perspective is based on the assumption that disturbed behavior is determined mainly be altered brain functioning. Psychiatric disorder is viewed as a disease. Neurobiologists express a belief that psychiatric syndromes may very well be composed of different pathophysiological processes and that some disorders are entirely attributable to altered neurochemistry. The genetic environmentalists hold that a biological or physiological defect is a necessary condition for mental illness and that psychiatric morbidity occurs only when persons with such inherited defects are faced with adverse circumstances that bring out their weaknesses. The genetically predisposed have nervous systems particularly vulnerable to the intense stimulation that social stress brings.

The biologic perspective is most consistent with the classical medical theory of disease which emphasizes organ pathology. The clinician adherent generally makes strong use of somatic treatments such as the phenothiazines, antidepressant medications and electro-convulsive therapy. The appropriate verbal approach is viewed as directive. This involves telling patients explicitly that they have an illness, explaining what steps must be taken for them to get better and providing support as required.

The Learning Perspective

According to the learning perspective, mental disorder is an example of abnormal behavior. This behavior reflects a learned, but persistent and maladaptive, response acquired in anxiety generating situations. The response is maladaptive because it is now manifest in situations where no objective threat exists. Overt symptoms are regarded as the proper focus of treatment since it is reasoned that they represent the problem and are not secondary manifestations of either disease or unconscious conflict.

Treatment approaches are based upon the idea that it is possible to develop schedules that weaken maladaptive responses and reinforce more adaptive behavior. The therapist determines the behavior to be modified, establishes the conditions under which the behavior occurs, determines the factors responsible for the behavior's persistence, selects the set of treatment conditions and arranges a retraining schedule. Behavioral techniques used to modify antecedent conditions include desensitization, reciprocal inhibition and condition avoidance. Those used to modify conditions that result from the behavior include positive and negative reinforcement, aversive conditioning and extinction.

Eclecticism

Up to this point, we have emphasized the association between particular illness perspectives and discrete therapeutic orientations. This relationship is depicted in figure 1-1. Thus, a somatotherapeutic orientation exists where a belief in the efficacy of somatic treatments is tied to a conviction that mental illness reflects organic disease of the brain or that disturbed behavior results from altered brain function. If a clinician views mental illness as a manifestation of intrapsychic conflict and makes extensive use of dynamically oriented expressive and exploratory verbal therapies, a psychotherapeutic orientation exists. The view that abnormal behavior is learned as a result of aversive stimuli coupled with the application of therapeutic techniques reinforcing adaptive and extinguishing maladaptive behaviors provides evidence of a behavioral orientation. Finally, where a belief that mental illness is caused by social and environmental factors dovetails with the use of a multiplicity of personal and social situation interventions as treatment vehicles, a sociotherapeutic orientation exists.

In actuality, practicing clinicians (Figure 1-2) blur the distinctions among illness perspectives and treatment orientations. This, in part, is a function of the inability of any single illness perspective to account satisfactorily for the wide range of psychopathologic and behaviorally maladaptive configurations with which the clinician must contend. It, in part, is also a function of clinical pragmatism. Society demands that a practitioner produce beneficial effects through the utilization of his skills. If a single treatment orientation does not consistently produce those effects, one would anticipate that practitioners might subscribe to a number of treatment orientations.

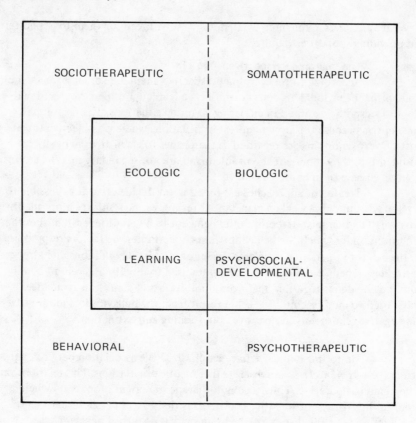

Figure 1-1. The Relationship between Illness Perspectives and Treatment Orientations

Selecting and combining aspects of various schools of thought or theories in an attempt to obtain a theoretical system that represents the best elements of any school is, by definition, eclecticism. In an applied field, this involves the use of any procedures, concepts and theoretical principles that seem appropriate for solving a particular problem, whether or not they form an integrated system. Thus, the pluralism that is so much a part of contemporary psychiatric practice can be viewed as a reflection of an eclecticism derived from the low level of confirmation currently enjoyed by psychiatric theory.

DIFFICULTIES IN PATIENT CARE EVALUATION

Some of the very issues that impinge upon practitioners, fostering the development of eclecticism, complicate the efforts of evaluators in assessing the quality of patient care. The difficulties begin with the need to separate the "mentally

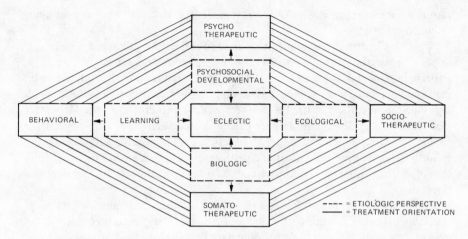

Figure 1-2. Eclectic and Non-Eclectic Treatment Orientations and Illness Perspectives

ill" from the population at large. The term "mentally ill" has been used to describe a host of phenomena ranging from schizophrenia through unhappiness to the tacit acceptance of an intolerable environment. As a result, estimates of the extent of illness vary considerably.

Plunkett and Gordon [4], in a review of prevalence studies undertaken prior to 1960, note that the percentage of population estimated to be mentally ill ranged from less than two percent to as much as 33 percent. The Dohrenwends [5], in examining 25 studies of untreated cases of psychological disorder, found prevalence rates reported in studies carried out after 1950 to be more than seven times those reported in studies in 1950 or earlier. These differences reflect variations in the criteria used to distinguish mental health from mental illness. Reported rates of illness tend to be lower when the definition is limited to the presence of a clearly established disabling condition than when the definition is broadened to encompass a wide range of problems in living. Attempts at circumventing this problem by defining the mentally ill operationally as identified patients, classified by clinicians according to standard diagnostic nomenclature, are also problematic. Significant questions have been raised about the reliability and validity of psychiatric diagnoses, and diagnoses per se have not always proven to be strong predictors of either choice of treatment or chance for recovery.[6-11]

The relative inability of the mental health field to generate conceptual models demonstrating fundamental relationships among etiology, cause of illness and response to treatment complicates the task of developing homogeneous patient populations or valid comparison groups. It also impedes the development of agreed upon standards to measure improvement in mental health status. As a result, the measures of change or improvement tend to be either construct-bound or construct-relative.

Construct-bound measures tend to reflect the values and assumptions implicit in a particular illness perspective or treatment orientation. While not entirely judgmental, the scales and indexes used often require that inferences be made and are somewhat biased. One example is the Health-Sickness Rating Scale developed by members of the Psychotherapy Research Project of the Menninger Foundation.[12] Seven criteria were balanced off to arrive at a single overall rating. The criteria included ability to function autonomously, seriousness of symptoms, subjective discomfort and distress, effect upon environment, utilization of abilities, quality of interpersonal relationships, and breadth and depth of interests.

Construct-relative measures attempt to minimize value-determined reporting by being non-inferential and atheoretical. They focus on objective phenomena with the intent of providing data that capture those aspects of the human condition that have psychological, social and clinical relevance. The data can be obtained from either self-administered or rate-administered forms. Frequently the instruments lend themselves to computer analysis. They may take the form of a symptom checklist or an inventory of social functioning.[13-15] While the data themselves need not be viewed as derivative of an illness perspective or treatment orientation, the information must still be interpreted and, therefore, is potentially subject to the same limits as measures embodying theoretical assumptions.

THREE APPROACHES FOR ASSESSING THE QUALITY OF PATIENT CARE

Despite the dilemmas outlined, a good deal of effort has been expended in developing evaluative strategies to facilitate the assessment of quality. Three approaches, in particular, have received considerable attention. Donabedian [16] refers to them as the review of structure, process and outcome. Zusman and Rieff [17] and Fox and Rappaport [18] explored the use of these approaches in mental health program evaluation. Let us examine briefly their application within the more limited context of patient care appraisal.

The Structural Approach

Structural approaches focus upon organizational aspects that have impact upon patient care, including personnel, facilities, equipment, information and record systems, formal organization and financing. In evaluating manpower, it is assumed that specified types and numbers of experts, qualified to deliver care, are necessary to ensure that quality care is given. The education and experience of the staff are investigated and used as an index of their professional competence. Sets of relationships within a program, professional time commit-

ments and organizational hierarchies, including areas of conflict of interest, can also be defined and evaluated to determine whether there are structural blocks preventing accomplishment of program goals.

While clearly seen as being related to the quality of patient care, structure is not equated with quality. Two basic assumptions underlie the use of a structural approach: (1) it is possible to identify what is "good" in terms of staff, physical structure and formal organization; (2) better care is more likely to be provided when better qualified staff, improved physical facilities and sounder fiscal and administrative procedures are applied. These assumptions make it possible to frame questions about quality in terms of organizational as well as clinical objectives. Thus, structural approaches can facilitate the evaluation of issues such as help-seeking behaviors, accessibility of services, continuity of care, productivity, efficiency and effectiveness.

Examples of structural approaches include Pugh and MacMahon's [19] study of continuity of care, McCaffree's [20] examination of the comparative efficiency of intensive versus custodial treatment, Ellsworth et al.'s [21] articulation of characteristics of productive as opposed to non-productive unit systems, Blackburn's [22] evaluation of factors affecting turnover rates in mental hospitals, Ullmann and Gurel's [23] demonstration of the influence that size and staffing have upon psychiatric hospital effectiveness, and the utilization studies of Tischler et al.[24,25] investigating questions related to help-seeking behaviors, accessibility and patterns of use found in populations served by catchment versus non-catchment oriented delivery systems.

The Evaluation of Process

Process evaluation makes use of criteria-oriented approaches and special studies to focus upon the activities of care-givers in the management of patients. The assumption underlying this form of evaluation is that the persons responsible for organizing and managing mental health services can generally agree upon what constitutes high quality treatment without continually monitoring outcome. In the appraisal of process one asks if the care rendered meets currently accepted standards. In essence, such appraisal provides feedback to insure that a patient care activity does what it claims.

Within the broad field of the evaluation of process, it is important to distinguish immediately two relatively different methodologies. One is to isolate the specific patterns of care by studying the aggregate characteristics of a large number of cases. The other involves individual case review.

In the first technique, the treatments prescribed for various diseases are reviewed, as are laboratory and other tests needed to establish diagnosis. They are compared with empirical or normative standards to determine whether the care rendered actually meets the standards of quality within the field. In the alternative technique, a committee, usually composed of clinicians, reviews the practice in given cases to see whether the patients have received care representa-

tive of the standards for contemporary practice. Such standards may be either implicit criteria, based on the committee's years of experience and general knowledge, or explicit criteria, often specific for diagnosis.

While criterion-oriented approaches have received extensive use in general medicine,[26–30] it has only been recently that a burgeoning interest has developed on the part of the mental health profession. Richman and Pinsker [31] describe a utilization review procedure for inpatient care involving the statement of therapeutic goals, predictions about the time required to reach these goals and the evaluation of care in terms of whether the goals have been met. The effectiveness of the procedure was suggested by the decrease in the number of patients with prolonged stays and the increase in the number of patients cared for. Zusman and Lawson described the use of an approach where a set of quantitative standards for quality assessment derived from expert opinion are applied to case review. The authors further recommend the use of direct observation as an alternative to record review. Their technique involves the selection and reporting of individual "critical incidents" by medical, nursing and clerical personnel. A critical incident is an observable activity that is complete enough to permit a reasonable determination that it will have an effect upon the quality of care. Once a large series of incidents are collected, it becomes possible to develop a quality scale based on the presence and/or absence of critical incidents.

Outcome Evaluation

Evaluation of outcome is a fundamentally different kind of review. Some direct measure of results is related to treatment given. Within this conceptual framework the qualifications of those rendering care, the structure of their organization and the extent to which they use acceptable methods can theoretically be disregarded in favor of appraising whether or not the desired results are achieved. In the evaluation of outcome, it is assumed that: (1) there is a strong concordance between societal and professional views of what end results are deemed desirable; (2) "good" results are brought about to a significant degree by good care; and, (3) those "good" results can be translated into indexes of success that reflect the effectiveness of the care-giving process. Thus, outcome evaluation provides the final evidence of whether care has been good or bad.

Examples of outcome evaluation are found in the work of Sheldon [32] and of Pasamanick et al.[33] Sheldon addressed himself to the question of how effective after-care was for discharged inpatients. Effectiveness was equated with the prevention of readmissions to hospital. The study sample included women between the ages of twenty and fifty-nine with a diagnosis of schizophrenia or depression. Eighty-nine successive patients were randomly assigned, upon discharge, to psychiatric after-care or to the care of a general practitioner. Within the psychiatric after-care group, patients were also randomly assigned to a day hospital or an outpatient clinic. The patients were followed for six months.

The readmission rate for after-care patients was 18 percent in contrast with 47 percent for those referred to general practitioners. No difference was found in readmissions between day hospital and outpatient clinic cases. Psychiatric aftercare was associated with a longer time spent under care during the follow-up period, but shorter subsequent hospitalizations. Pasamanick et al. explored the relative value of hospital versus home care for schizophrenic patients. One hundred fifty-two patients referred to a state hospital were randomly distributed among three groups: drug/home care; placebo/home care; hospital care. Home care treatment provided by public health nurses was compared with hospital treatment and home-care patients receiving medications were compared with home-care patients who received placebos. Patients were involved in the study from six to thirty months. During the period of study, 77 percent of the drug/home-care group required no hospitalization in contrast with 34 percent of those receiving a placebo. Members of the control groups treated in hospital required more frequent rehospitalization after return to the community than patients treated on drugs at home from the start. Data on psychological and social functioning collected after six, eighteen and twenty-four months revealed considerable improvement in all groups by the sixth month, scant improvement thereafter and no superiority between one or another form of treatment.

THE PSYCHIATRIC UTILIZATION REVIEW AND EVALUATION (PURE) PROJECT

While the reviews of structure, process and outcome each contribute to our understanding of the quality of patient care, it is clear that they are interdependent. Appropriate structure increases the probability of good care which, in turn, enhances the likelihood of successful outcome. One would suspect, therefore, that the information obtained from an evaluative system that synthesized the approaches would be greater than the mere sum of the three. This was essentially the conclusion reached by members of the Psychiatric Utilization Review and Evaluation (PURE) Project.

Supported under a grant and contract with the National Institute of Mental Health, the project represented a collaborative venture by members of the Connecticut Mental Health Center and the Departments of Psychiatry, Epidemiology and Public Health, and Sociology of Yale University. Members of the Administrative Science Department at Yale, and the Multi-State Information System (MSIS), and the Connecticut Utilization and Patient Information Statistical System (CUPIS) acted as consultants.

The projects aims were:

1. To develop a model of utilization review suitable for mental health centers which would show the utility and the interrelationship of the various components of the utilization review system; that is, criteria for adequacy of care,

mechanisms for selecting cases for review, follow-up studies and special studies such as epidemiologic examination of patients to determine their representativeness of the areas from which they come.

2. To determine the best means to construct explicit standards for adequacy of care through the use of different approaches by panels of clinicians such as diagnosis, symptom, developmental epoch, or institutional process.

3. To delineate the strategic patient characteristics for first-screening process in utilization review, based on norms as developed by panels and on the detailed analysis of patterns of care.

4. To construct mechanisms for case selection, based on the combinations of patient characteristics specified above.

5. To implement the components of the review mechanisms in the Connecticut Mental Health Center.

6. To construct a set of components for a patient care evaluation system for possible use in other centers.

7. To document the problems involved in setting up a model for utilization review in psychiatry.

Thus, in brief, there were four major phases to the project:

1. The development of criteria for evaluation and mechanisms for case selection;
2. The testing of criteria and mechanisms;
3. The implementation of a system of patient care evaluation; and,
4. The testing of such a system and its export to other centers.

In chapter 2, Myers presents a more detailed description of the organization and evolution of the PURE Project. An important side effect of the work, however, was a growing awareness that the process of utilization review, properly defined, could be used as a technique to measure several dimensions of overall program effectiveness, including the end results of various modalities of care. The dilemma was how best to link the evaluative endeavor to the actual delivery of service.

A CONTEXTUAL MODEL FOR PATIENT CARE EVALUATION

A general systems perspective can help to elaborate potential relationships between the delivery and the evaluation of patient care. If one views a mental health service program as a set of elements or parts which have a definable organization or interrelationship, then it can be depicted as a complex social system in constant interaction with its environment. Within a given population, individuals at risk are either referred to or seek out the services of the program. Entry is through an evaluation subsystem whence the applicant may be discharged back into the community, referred to another mental health treatment program, returned to the referring agent or agency, or be transferred to the program's treatment subsystem. At time of discharge from treatment, the patient reenters the community and, indeed, may represent an important part of the population at risk with a likelihood of subsequent recycling through the system or direct reentry into the treatment subsystem.

As figure 1–3 illustrates, such a systems perspective provides a fulcrum for organizing an evaluative endeavor to facilitate a synthesis of structural, process and outcome approaches. The system's inputs take on a variety of forms such as personnel, time, money, information and actual and potential users that lend themselves to structural analyses. A system's through-put includes programs and subprograms structured to fulfill task requirements. Since through-put involves both technologic and managerial dimensions of organizational processes, it can best be assessed through a combination of structural and process approaches. Similarly, a system's output takes on a variety of forms such as products, profits and satisfactions that lend themselves to both structural and outcome analysis. The former addresses questions of comparative cost, efficiency and cost-benefit; the latter, questions related to changes in those served.

While, admittedly, the formulation offered is somewhat simplistic, it does allow for a conceptual approximation of patient care evaluation to the actual delivery of mental health services. Before attempting to implement an evaluative endeavor of this nature, however, it is extremely important to insure the availability of an adequate data base. Brenner and Myers address themselves to this question in chapter 3. After presenting a historical overview of the evolution of data requirements, they proceed to detail the types of data necessary for an attempt to link patient care evaluation to a comprehensive model for the delivery of mental health services. Once the requirements are stated, they present supporting evidence for the utility of the basic data list and move to a consideration of its value in facilitating both utilization review and patient care evaluation.

In chapter 4, Henisz, Tischler and Myers elaborate on the application of the data base in evaluating input. Emphasis is placed upon the use of epidemiologic and ecologic studies, both to clarify issues related to the demand versus the need for service and to evaluate help-seeking behaviors, patterns of utilization and questions related to the availability and accessibility of care.

Chapters 5 through 7 shift attention to the evaluation of system throughput. Tischler begins chapter 5 by focusing on the operational use of criteria to define quality. The quality of care is segregated into three components—appropriateness, adequacy and effectiveness—and general approaches for formulating such criteria are expounded. After presenting examples of derived criteria, the advantages and limitations of a criterion-oriented approach are examined. In chapter 6, Goldblatt builds upon the more general discussion of standard development to detail various processes that facilitate the transformation of indexes and predetermined criteria into mechanisms for evaluating patient care. Brauer and Riedel proceed, in chapter 7, to an extensive discussion of individual case review, methods of selecting cases for review, and techniques

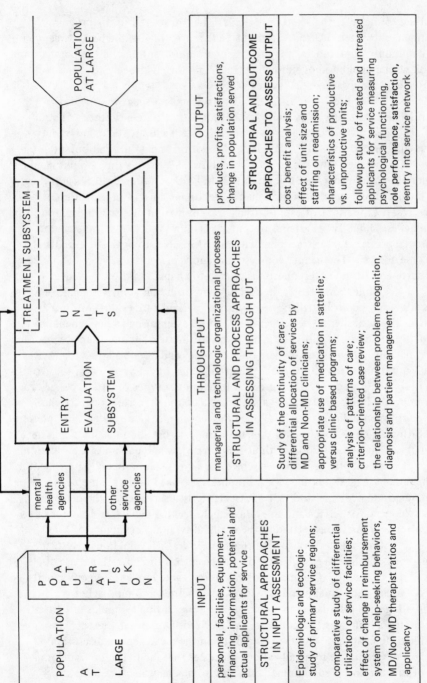

Figure 1-3.   Patient Care Evaluation within the Context of a Service Delivery Model

for developing statistical mechanisms that enhance case selection. An evaluation of the various methods and techniques is presented.

The focus then shifts from the use of criterion-oriented approaches in throughput analysis to a consideration of the role that special studies and follow-up studies play in patient care evaluation. In chapter 8, Weissman and Paykel provide an operational definition of "special study" before going into a detailed exposition of its potential use. The transformation from potential to actual is made through the presentation of a series of special studies undertaken in order to gain a firmer understanding of a particular clinical problem, suicidal behavior. Data are set forth illustrating the value of special study for developing and testing criteria, as well as analyzing, in depth, discrete problems related to the process of care. Schwartz and Myers restate these themes in relation to follow-up study (chapter 9). They advance the proposition that follow-up can become a routine part of an evaluative endeavor when carefully planned to coincide with the use of a standardized record-keeping system. Particular attention is placed upon overcoming methodologic problems encountered while conducting research in the natural setting. A detailed description of follow-up study is presented to demonstrate how patient care evaluation is facilitated through the generation of palpable data on a system's output that allows for a determination of outcome and its relationship to treatment.

Having articulated an approach to patient care evaluation that dovetails with an operational model for the delivery of mental health services, one must still contend with issues of applicability. In chapter 10, Cytrynbaum looks beyond the realm of patient care and explores the utility of a criteria-oriented approach in the evaluation of indirect services. The basic question raised is whether the approach is applicable for monitoring the quality of complex, non-clinical interventions such as community organization, program consultation and case consultation. A conceptual overview is presented, together with preliminary work in translating the constructs into operational measures and developing the requisite instrumentation. In the final chapter, the issue of applicability is addressed from the perspective of feasibility. Goldblatt, Henisz and Tischler draw upon the PURE project's experience with a number of mental health centers attempting to initiate a system of utilization review. They explore issues related to the appropriate organizational framework for an evaluative endeavor, set forth recommendations for implementing a patient care evaluation and utilization review system, and underline difficulties to be anticipated with any attempt at institutionalizing patient care assessment.

OVERVIEW

By adopting the position that the evaluation of patient care encompasses utilization review and is a basic component of program evaluation, we have located the evaluative endeavor as an integral part of the mental health delivery system. Our emphasis upon the contextual relatedness of both the evaluation and the delivery of service is intended to contest a view of evaluation as either encapsulated from or unrelated to program.

Service programs usually develop because of perceived needs. Goals are then promulgated by the agency responsible for filling the needs. Management develops a program consistent with the goals. An evaluation group is assigned the task of determining whether the program is, in actuality, meeting the goals. The evaluative task involves translating the goals into operational terms, identifying proper criteria for use in measuring success, determining and explaining the degree of success achieved and recommending further program activity.

The inclusion of feedback and program modification as core elements of an evaluative enterprise assumes that programs are, by nature, evolutionary; modification of program is likely to be required to facilitate the attainment of predetermined goals; the objectives themselves may well require periodic review and, at times, explication or even reformulation. Thus, the evaluative endeavor must of necessity be in constant interaction with program and agents of the program; for its worth derives from a capacity not only to measure achievement but also to yield information useful in decision making.

Ideally, the program should be evaluated on the basis of its success in attaining ultimate goals—for example, a decrease in the prevalence of drug addiction in the community after instituting a comprehensive drug abuse program. Since the full impact of a program is, most typically, either visible only after a considerable time lag or not readily accessible to direct and easy observation, much evaluation focuses upon intermediate results (e.g., the number of addicts enrolled in a detoxification program) or short-term outcome (e.g., the number of addicts drug free six months after discharge).

Since the feedback and recommendations for program modification related to ultimate objectives are frequently extrapolated from data measuring intermediate results, strains are often introduced in the relationship between the evaluator-as-commentator and other agents of the program. In a field where the measurement of success involves difficult methodologic and ideologic issues and a dearth of effective outcome studies exists, the need to offer formulations that must rely somewhat upon inference is bound to generate a degree of conflict. With proper attention to the breadth of material to evaluate and to the many levels of feedback necessary, however, a systematic approach to evaluation should result both in the clarification of conceptually clouded issues and in enhanced quality of care.

Chapter Two

Psychiatric Utilization Review and Evaluation Project

Donald C. Riedel
Jerome K. Myers
Gary L. Tischler

In June of 1969, the Psychiatric Utilization Review and Evaluation (PURE) Project was begun in New Haven as a collaborative undertaking by members of the Connecticut Mental Health Center and the Departments of Epidemiology and Public Health, Psychiatry and Sociology of Yale University. A working arrangement was established immediately with the Multi-State Information System (MSIS) and two years later with three additional mental health centers: Area B Mental Health Center, Washington, D.C.; Erich Lindermann Mental Health Center, Boston; and Rockland County Community Mental Health Center, Pomona, New York. Additionally, members of the Administrative Sciences Department at Yale and the Connecticut Utilization and Patient Information System (CUPIS) served as consultants.

Because of the large number of individuals and organizations associated with the research, a central planning committee was formed to set policy and coordinate the broad range of activities being undertaken. This committee included the five principal co-investigators, the project coordinators and the director of the schizophrenia field study. Disciplines represented were nursing, psychiatry, public health and sociology.

Under this planning committee's jurisdiction, the project activities were organized and coordinated during its four major phases: (1) the development of criteria for evaluation and mechanisms for case selection, (2) the testing of criteria and mechanisms and evaluation of quality of patient care, (3) the development and implementation of a system of patient care evaluation and/or utilization review and (4) the testing of such a system and its export to other centers. Although the four phases represent an approximate chronology of the project's major activities, the establishment and specific undertakings of the various groups described below were not necessarily limited to any one phase. The planning of a number of field studies concerned mainly with testing of criteria was begun, for example, as soon as the project began. Similarly, the clinical panels both developed and tested criteria, and the data group participated in all phases of the study. The outline of the project's structure is shown in figure 2-1. (See appendix A for a listing of all persons associated with the project.)

THE DEVELOPMENT OF CRITERIA FOR EVALUATION AND MECHANISMS FOR CASE SELECTION

The Clinical Panels

At the beginning of the project, peer group panels were formed for the purpose of developing criteria for patient care evaluation and assessing their feasibility, reliability and validity through ongoing research. This approach was based on the general principle that criteria should be developed by peer groups composed primarily, but not exclusively, of clinicians. Thus three of the four panels organized was headed by a Connecticut Mental Health Center (CMHC) clinician; the fourth was chaired by a psychologist. While the panels included psychiatric clinicians from CMHC, attention was given to insure participation by others (e.g., social workers, nurses, and faculty within the Yale Department of Psychiatry) who were not on the staff of CMHC. In addition, nonclinicians (e.g., social scientists and public health researchers) were participants in all panels.

Figure 2-1.   Structure of the PURE Project

Central Planning Committee

A. The development of criteria for evaluation and mechanisms for case selection.
   1. The clinical panels
      a. Schizophrenia
      b. Suicide
      c. Adolescence
      d. Intake
   2. The data group
   3. Connecticut Utilization and Patient Information System (CUPIS) and Yale Department of Administrative Science Consultants
B. The testing of criteria and mechanisms and evaluation of quality of patient care.
   1. Schizophrenia field study
   2. Outpatient field study
   3. Epidemiology survey
   4. Indirect care studies
C. The development and implementation of a system of patient care evaluation and/or utilization review.
   1. Program Information and Analysis Section (PIAS), Connecticut Mental Health Center (CMHC)
   2. The Multi-State Information System for Psychiatric Patients (MSIS)
D. The testing of such a system and its export to other centers.
   1. Erich Lindemann Mental Health Center, Boston
   2. Area B Mental Health Center, Washington, D.C.
   3. Rockland Community Mental Health Center, Pomona, New York
   4. Connecticut Mental Health Center, New Haven, Connecticut

Each panel was charged with generating a research approach to its task. The panels were encouraged to formulate initial criteria on the basis of their own clinical experience and their review of the literature. At the same time, liaison was established between each panel and the data group (described below) to allow in-depth analysis of the large body of data available on the 1968-69 cohort of CMHC patients. The initial charge to each panel was quite broad, and the operational guidelines quite flexible, in order to elicit fresh perspectives on method of approach.

After considerable discussion concerning clinical areas to be reviewed by the panels, it was agreed that evaluation based exclusively on the American Psychiatric Association diagnostic classification was inadequate. Therefore, four panels were selected representing alternative approaches to defining patient-care problems. These areas were:

Schizophrenia. Schizophrenia represents a defined diagnostic group which has major importance in contemporary psychiatry. Alternative treatments are available and efforts at secondary and tertiary prevention have been defined.

Suicide. Suicide represents a widespread and dramatic psychosocial behavior. Patients who attempt suicide represent a population at risk. Intervention programs have preventive potential, especially since there are well-defined outcomes (i.e., repeated suicide attempts or actual self-induced death).

Adolescence. Adolescence represents a psychosocial and psychosexual developmental period. As a panel topic, it was chosen to allow a developmental approach to a social group undergoing rapid social change. Concepts from sociology, education, developmental psychology, psychoanalysis and ego psychology contribute to an evaluation of the patient's relationship to family, school system and community.

Intake. Intake is defined in terms of a systems approach and an institutional process. It taps into the process by which referred clients and applicants become "patients." Developing criteria for intake is especially relevant and timely because of the increasing rate at which community psychiatric facilities are being utilized, necessitating rapid evaluation and emergency care. This panel provided a linkage between the CMHC and the emergency service of the Yale–New Haven Hospital, which, although it is architecturally and administratively separate, is an integral part of the mental health care system.

It is important to note that each of the panels was expected, after developing guidelines, to test them for feasibility, reliability and validity. This involved some research endeavors by each of the panels. For this purpose the panels were provided, during the second year of the project, with research assistants and programming time as well as any necessary ancillary personnel within budgetary limits.

The *schizophrenia panel* first developed a definition of schizophrenia that could be used both in prospective studies and for chart review. Following extensive literature review, theoretical discussions and pilot work, a checklist and scoring system were developed and tested. In order to explore the reliability and validity of the checklist and scoring system, a study of the records of over 670 schizophrenic and non-schizophrenic patients was undertaken. The Yale Schizophrenia Index was developed from this work. Once this basic work was completed, guidelines for patient care evaluation were developed.

The *panel on suicide* developed criteria for six evaluation and treatment decisions: (1) what kind of patients ought to be evaluated for suicidal potential; (2) what ought that evaluation consist of; (3) which suicidal patients ought to be hospitalized; (4) who ought to be offered outpatient treatment; (5) who ought to have general medical or surgical treatment; (6) who should be compelled to accept treatment. The panel also made an interview study of a sample of persons who had been admitted to the emergency room of the Yale-New Haven Medical Center for suicidal attempts or gestures.

The *panel on adolescence* developed a set of guidelines for adolescent clinical care and criteria for chart review. It paid particular attention to the chief complaint section of the clinical chart which was frequently unclear and seemed to indicate faulty communication between the patient and clinician. Accordingly, the panel developed a questionnaire to study this confusion and administered it to a sample of 100 adolescents and their clinicians over a four-month period. A modified form of the chief complaint check list was administered to 100 high school adolescents who were not patients to determine to what extent the problems that patients feel bring them to treatment at CMHC are reflected in the general population. Finally, a study of forty discharged patients was conducted to obtain their impressions about clinical care.

The *intake panel* was concerned with both patient care and program evaluation. It adopted three perspectives on the intake process: epidemiological, institutional and clinical (individual patient care). In addition to developing broad guidelines for patient care evaluation and utilization review, the panel participated in the epidemiological study described later in this chapter.

Although the panels experienced varying degrees of success in developing criteria, it is clear that the exact goal of criteria development was related to the particular approach to be adopted. Guidelines for individual case review were developed most efficiently by panels based on a medical diagnosis (schizophrenia) or modified to some degree by the inclusion of symptom complexes such as suicide. On the other hand, the adolescent and intake panels were more successful in developing guidelines for overall program evaluation, including the relationships between a mental health center and other community agencies.

The Data Group
Basic to all of the activities of the project was the development of techniques for data collection and analysis. Therefore, a data group was imme-

diately established under the direction of a sociologist-statistician. The group included six other members and represented specialists in data analysis, computer programming, psychiatric administration and psychiatric therapy.

The initial task of the group was to undertake a retrospective analysis of the data available in 1968–69 patient records at CMHC in order to provide preliminary material on patterns of care analysis. This material was used for hypothesis testing by the panels and for developing statistically normative patterns of care. Such patterns served as a baseline to measure actual care against the type of treatment recommended by the panels according to their criteria. Discrepancies between the two served as focuses for further discussion, refinement of criteria and eventual evaluation of treatment.

A second task of the data group was the design, construction and testing of a data system for psychiatric utilization review in a community mental health center and the provision of pertinent data from this information system to expert panels and specialized study groups involved in the initial utilization review effort. This function was extremely important since utilization review is well-nigh impossible without an adequate data system. The data group provided direct assistance to the CMHC administration in preparation of data from administration reports, thus demonstrating the value of a well-functioning and ordered data system.

The data group also provided liaison with other groups in the development of a data system. It provided assistance to the records and information department of CMHC in developing their records and in working with the Multi-State Information System (MSIS) in helping the center to computerize records. In this connection, the data group assisted in the development of additional forms necessary to obtain information of importance for case review (e.g., the development of a contact form which would indicate the type of therapy, the number of therapy sessions and duration of therapy). It also collaborated with MSIS throughout the project in their joint efforts related to data systems at the other three cooperating mental health centers and with CUPIS in developing computerized techniques for case selection and patterns of care analyses. Finally, the data group was responsible for the management of computer services for the PURE project, including the provision of such services and technical expertise to the panels and specialized study groups.

CUPIS and Yale Department of Administrative Science Consultants

Prior to the start of the PURE Project, members of the Departments of Administrative Science and Epidemiology and Public Health at Yale and the Connecticut Utilization and Patient Information System (CUPIS) had developed a model of utilization review for short-term general hospitals—Basic Utilization Review Program (BURP). This system included case selection, problem-specific criteria (guidelines) for case evaluation, chart-abstracting techniques to facilitate the review process, and system-monitoring and feedback mechanisms to insure efficacious case selection and appraisal. Riedel was the director of this research group, and the logistical aspects of BURP and the objectives of each of the components had important implications for psychiatric utilization review. Therefore, other persons affiliated with that group were called upon for consultation in techniques of case selection, criteria development and other aspects of a utilization review system as the PURE Project got underway. These persons were also extremely helpful in developing computer techniques for analyses of patterns of care as that phase of the project progressed.

TESTING OF CRITERIA AND MECHANISMS AND EVALUATION OF QUALITY OF PATIENT CARE

Three major projects were concerned mainly with testing criteria and evaluating quality of patient care: the schizophrenia field study, the outpatient field study, the epidemiologic survey, and the indirect care studies. The clinical panels and the program information and analysis section (PIAS) of CMHC also tested criteria, but their primary functions were respectively criteria development and the implementation of a system of patient care evaluation.

In the studies described below the concept of patient care evaluation is extended beyond the isolated institutional stay to include the complex of care pertaining to a given episode of illness. In addition, these studies deal with program evaluation as well as individual patient care and utilization review.

Schizophrenia Field Study

The primary aims of the schizophrenia field study were to evaluate outcome of treatment for schizophrenia, to document treatment patterns and to relate these patterns to treatment outcome. More specifically, this follow-up study: (1) examined and compared patient characteristics and treatment methods as observed in various treatment settings; (2) determined the differential impact of various treatment modalities and their institutional contexts upon long term outcome in terms of social adjustment, role performance and psychiatric symptomatology and (3) determined the impact of intervening social stresses upon outcome.

The sample consisted of 132 people who were treated as inpatients and discharged to the community from six treatment units offering varied types of psychiatric care. In order to establish uniform diagnostic criteria for inclusion in the sample across the six treatment units being studied, the Yale Schizophrenic Index was used to select persons for the study. Patients, along with a family member, were interviewed one and one-half to four years after discharge, depending on the availability of cases on each unit. In addition, data were collected from written records and staff interviews. The results of this study demonstrated the differential impact of treatment, sociodemographic and natural history variables upon different outcome measures.

Outpatient Field Study

In 1968 a group at Yale accepted a contract from NIMH to gather behavioral ratings on a sample of outpatients at CMHC and to elaborate a design for the study of outpatients, especially around issues of intake and evaluation.

Persons who applied for treatment as outpatients at CMHC from October 1968 to June 1969 and who kept their first appointment were selected randomly for study. They were interviewed before intake on their expectations regarding treatment and after intake on symptomatology, social adjustment and attitude toward both the intake just completed and the clinician who undertook it. This involved 335 patients. Additional data were collected through interviews with a relative or close friend; questionnaires completed by clinicians on their views of their patients' symptoms, social and interpersonal behavior, expectations and personality attributes; and the measurement of clinicians' personalities and treatment ideologies through various scales.

In analyzing the data, clinical practice on the catchmented service—Hill West Haven (HWH)—was compared with practices on the General Clinical Division (GCD) in order to determine if any differences resulted from catchmenting as a means of organizing the delivery of services.

Epidemiological Survey

This study compared the use of mental health services by catchmented and non-catchmented populations served by the Hill West Haven and General Clinical Division of CMHC. Since a straightforward comparison of catchmented and non-catchmented populations could be misleading because of socioeconomic, ethnic and cultural differences of the area being surveyed, controls were introduced to insure homogeneity in the populations in terms of a group of independent variables that have been shown to correlate with the utilization of mental health services. Inner city populations were matched on a block-group by block-group basis and suburban populations on a census-tract by census-tract basis, utilizing data obtained from a special United States Census conducted in New Haven in 1967 on the following criteria: (1) total population; (2) proportion of non-white population; (3) overcrowding index—the percentage of housing units with 1.01 or more persons per room; (4) socioeconomic status index and (5) the normal family life index—the percentage of children under 18 living with both parents. The matched populations included 44,463 residents from the catchmented area and 45,471 from the non-catchmented area. These populations served as the baselines for calculations of utilization rates for mental health services and for comparisons of various patient populations.

Between July 1, 1969, and June 30, 1970, all admissions to the catchmented service (HWH), to the general service (GCD) and to the emergency room (ER) were recorded. Sociodemographic and clinical data were obtained from admission forms and patient charts in order to determine the differences in services and patient characteristics resulting from catchmenting as a method of organizing mental health services.

THE IMPLEMENTATION OF A SYSTEM OF
PATIENT CARE EVALUATION

The implementation, as well as part of the development, of a system of utilization review and patient care evaluation was carred out at CMHC. CMHC, financed and sponsored jointly by the state of Connecticut, the federal government and Yale University, is located near the center of New Haven and is part of the Yale–New Haven medical complex. The major divisions of CMHC include a general clinical division with in- and outpatient services, a catchmented service and an inpatient research unit. The mental health center has close relationships with other parts of the Yale–New Haven medical complex, especially its emergency services which serve as a source of intake.

During the implementation phase, the Multi-State Information System (MSIS) was especially helpful, although this group was associated with the project from the beginning.

Program Information and Analysis Section, CMHC

From the beginning of the study, the PURE Project worked closely with the Program Information and Analysis Section (PIAS) of CMHC in developing and testing criteria for utilization review based upon the work of the four clinical panels. The *Chart Review Checklist for Psychiatric Utilization Review*, which was later tested in other centers as well, grew out of the joint effort of the two groups. It consists of a compilation of criteria about the adequacy of intake/evaluation and of treatment as recorded in a chart.

Once a system of utilization review and patient care evaluation was developed, it was introduced into CMHC through the PIAS unit. A center-wide utilization review and patient care evaluation committee was established to implement the system. The utilization review process itself includes three successive stages or levels of review which differ according to the number of charts, the expertise with which review is accomplished and the extent and quality of information reviewed. These three levels of review are reflected in the format of the checklist.

The first-level review is applied to charts on all patients admitted to treatment at a mental health center and is accomplished by records room personnel. The goal of this level of review is to establish the completeness of the information contained in the chart. Charts found not to meet the minimal standards of completeness as required by the checklist are returned to the attending clinician for completion.

The second-level review is accomplished on samples of charts selected for intensive review. This stage is carried out by professional non-clinical personnel under the supervision of a psychiatrist. The goals of this level of review are to establish the adequacy of the information contained in the chart for clinical review and to establish whether or not the treatment, reflected in the information included in the chart, meets the criteria of good patient care set forth in the checklist. This level of review is not intended to establish adequacy of clinical care but only conformity to model standards of care represented in the criteria. Judgment of adequacy of care is the function of clinical level review.

The third-level review includes all charts found not to conform to the criteria incorporated in the checklist and a certain proportion of other charts, randomly selected from those reviewed in earlier stages by expert clinicians of a mental health center's utilization review committee. The goals of this level of review are to establish the adequacy of the patient care provided, in those instances where the standards prescribed in the checklist were not followed, and to provide continuing testing of the adequacy of the criteria in the checklist to discriminate adequate and inadequate patient care at earlier levels of review.

The Multi-State Information System for Psychiatric Patients

MSIS is a comprehensive, computer-based system designed to provide both automated clinical information and a management support system for patients in participating facilities. Currently, Connecticut, Hawaii, Massachusetts, New York, Rhode Island, Vermont and the District of Columbia are linked to the system, which has its headquarters and its computer at Rockland State Hospital, New York. The system is designed to follow the patient through all phases of psychiatric service by utilizing information normally gathered in the admission, treatment and discharge processes. Data are recorded on preprinted forms at the individual psychiatric and mental health agencies and then entered into the central file at Rockland.

At the start of the PURE Project a significant amount of effort was spent merging the data system of CMHC with that of MSIS. The two groups also collaborated in developing new forms to be used at CMHC and the other mental health centers involved in the project. The MSIS system was used for securing data for patterns of care analysis in the initial phase of criteria development. Later, its facilities were used to select cases for utilization review and patient care evaluation in the four participating mental health centers.

TESTING THE SYSTEM OF PATIENT CARE EVALUATION AND UTILIZATION REVIEW AND EXPORT TO OTHER CENTERS

In order to test the system of patient care evaluation and utilization review, we included three community mental health centers in addition to CMHC. To be included, the centers had to be within a day's travel from New Haven—because of the need for frequent visits to the centers by the PURE staff—be a member of MSIS so that all would be part of the same data system, and be representative of a range of centers in terms of location, university affiliation and source of funding.

The three centers which joined in the collaborative effort in the third year of the project included: Erich Lindemann Mental Health Center, Boston—a Harvard University affiliated center similar to CMHC in many respects; Area B Mental Health Center, Washington, D.C.—a federal mental health center in a large inner city area; and Rockland County Community Mental Health Center, Pomona, New York—a suburban-rural center not connected with a university or state system and locally controlled. These three centers plus CMHC were the locations for the final testing and modification of the review and evaluation system.

The objectives of the joint collaboration between the mental health centers and PURE were to implement the utilization review model developed by PURE and CMHC, to further modify it according to the needs of the various centers, and to provide materials which would enable us to evaluate the various utilization review mechanisms which were established.

More specifically, all four mental health centers agreed: (1) to establish a functioning utilization review mechanism; (2) to provide the PURE Project with a description of the objectives, composition and functioning of the mechanism responsible for utilization review and patient care evaluation activity in the center; (3) to provide the PURE Project with any reports and minutes of this activity that would be done routinely as part of the utilization review process (including the selection of committee members), with a documentation reflecting the modifications made in the checklist used for case evaluation, and with the rationale for making the revisions; (4) to allow the PURE Project access to an extract of the data base stored in the MSIS system for patients treated from January 1971 to the termination of the project; and (5) to apply the checklists to individual cases and to provide the PURE Project with completed checklists.

For its part, PURE provided the following for the centers: (1) a checklist to be used in the utilization review process covering the admission, treatment and discharge stages of patient care; (2) selection criteria and programming for use of selection criteria of medical records so that patients can be selected from the MSIS data base according to these criteria; (3) pattern analysis and its programming based on current and future data; and (4) results of the checklist analysis with interpretive comments.

Individual patient identification information was deleted from all material from the centers and was not available to PURE. Specifically, this included: patient's name, case number, social security number and exact street address. Since PURE required some method of identifying individual patient records, dummy codes were established and assigned to patient records. The originating center retained the listing of the dummy codes and was the sole party to have access to this listing. Use of the data were in accordance with state and District of Columbia rules and regulations pertaining to research use of mental health data. Reporting of data was restricted to feedback to participating centers, NIMH and MSIS, unless other specific arrangements were made with the centers in writing.

Data from the centers were used to develop selection criteria for identification of cases for utilization review as well as effective review checklists for use by individual utilization review committees for case evaluation. The analyses and interpretations contained in the reports of the project preserved the anonymity of both the individual centers and the patients served by those centers. The emphasis of the reports was upon the development of a technique of analysis rather than upon the actual value of the discrete variables. The release of the analysis was dependent upon the review of the participants.

In This Chapter: the structure of the PURE Project has been described in terms of its four major phases. There was much overlap in the activities of the various groups, and many staff members participated in the activities of several groups. Work frequently progressed at an uneven pace, and coordination of the endeavors of such a large number of professionals was at times difficult. On more than one occasion the central planning committee questioned the feasibility of its undertaking. However, by the end of the project not only had most of the original goals been reached, but many new ones had been developed and met. In the following chapters the results are presented.

Chapter Three

Data and Data Systems
for Patient Care Evaluation

M. Harvey Brenner
Jerome K. Myers

Basic to any system of utilization review is some type of data system, whether or not it is computerized. The systems we utilized were all computerized and had many advantages for that reason, but data systems need not necessarily be computerized to conduct utilization review and patient care evaluation. Regardless of the type of data system, however, the clinical record is basic to any review process. It provides crucial information not only for individual case evaluation but also for management and administrative policy for the entire treatment agency.

Starting with individual cases, the clinical record should include four types of information in order to document the treatment process. The first is a statement of the patient's problem or the reason he contacted the institution for treatment. The statement of the problem is traditionally presented in the form of the *chief complaint*, indication of signs or symptoms, history of present illness, any defined life situations requiring assistance, social functioning and clinical diagnosis. Second, it is assumed that the *plan for treatment* is directly related to the clinical statement of the patient's problem(s). Where this relationship is not present or is unclear, a statement of rationale is pertinent. Each major feature of the treatment plan should be recorded, including types of therapy, interval, periodicity and dosage (or amount of time per psychotherapy session). Third, the *treatment* should be fully recorded—types of therapy, individuals responsible, actual length of treatment, and periodicity and dosages (or psychotherapeutic interval). Where the actual course of treatment departs significantly from the treatment plan or from clinical norms, a rationale should be given. Fourth, indicators of the patient's progress in relation to the treatment received are usually summarized in the form of *progress notes*. These notes are of considerable importance as evidence that the process of clinical evaluation was possible and that the patient's progress was examined.

Clinical records are also important for administrative purposes. In the aggregate they provide information on the sociodemographic and clinical characteristics of the patient population which may identify certain groups by age, diagnostic categories, etc. requiring special attention or services. Clinical records also provide data on patterns of care (utilization of institutional facilities and points of referral to and from the institution). The institution may be under- or overrepresented by specific referral sources or may be referring an unusually high (or low) proportion of patients to outside facilities (e.g., general hospitals, state mental hospitals, halfway houses). In general, points of referral to and from the institution are important data for understanding the significance of the institution within the spectrum of patient care. Finally, the information contained in clinical records allows the administrator to know who is being served and whether his institution's program is providing equitable care and efficient service. It is important to recognize that a great variety of sociodemographic factors may produce skewed utilization patterns. Such a skewing, for example, may be peculiar to the population covered by the institution and may involve, among other factors, age, sex, ethnicity, residential area, marital status and education.

Despite the importance of clinical records, there is great variation in their content, both within and between psychiatric facilities. This variation arises from several sources. Knowledge of the etiology of most major mental disorders is minimal, and there is only an imprecise understanding of the relative effectiveness of many psychiatric therapies. It is not surprising, therefore, that clinicians may disagree as to which data are appropriate and should be recorded. In fact, the very mechanism of peer review may serve to inhibit comparable recording among clinicians because of professional disagreement as to appropriate procedures. Additional difficulties may occur where treatment procedures are subject to administrative policies which conflict with specific objectives in the management of individual cases. Such administrative influences on patient care may not be consistent with the clinical rationale for either choice or conduct of therapy. There may therefore appear to be a lack of logical fit between the statement of a patient's problem and the therapy given as indicated in the clinical record. In such cases, it may not be possible to infer from the record the actual reasons for the course of therapy utilized.

Nevertheless, in order to carry out utilization review certain basic information must be contained in clinical records:

1. Identifying and sociodemographic data (e.g., name, age, sex, race, marital status, education, area of residence)
2. Source of referral to the institution
3. Problem (or diagnosis), and rationale (e.g., signs, symptoms) where not inferrable from statement of the problem
4. Treatment plan, with rationale if not directly inferrable
5. Treatment course, with rationale if different from plan
6. Statement(s) of patient's progress (as related to treatment)

7. Patient's condition on discharge
8. Reason for discharge of patient
9. Place to which patient was referred from the institution

METHODS FOR STANDARDIZATION OF DATA

Given the variability of clinical psychiatric data, methods for the standardization of data considered necessary by professional consensus must be developed. During the past twenty years, particularly the last decade, significant technological advances in such standardization have been made in four major areas: (1) the development of standardized forms for rapid recording of data pertinent to psychiatric evaluation; (2) experimentation with restructured forms of the medical record, especially with problem-oriented recording; (3) the development of scales for the measurement of mental status; and (4) computer-based recording, storage and retrieval systems as well as methods of linkage to additional data sources.

Each of these developments has direct application to utilization review. They all involve recording and processing information relevant to the evaluation of patient care. The technologies of data processing assure standardization, and therefore comparability, of the sequence and rationale of patient care among clinicians and facilities. These developments also make possible the aggregation and sorting of relatively large bodies of data recording experience with patient care. Given such data sources, it becomes possible to screen both retrospectively and concurrently for normative and unusual patterns of care, with the additional benefit of testing for statistical significance. Once identified via screening procedures, the problems of utilization can be probed more incisively and in greater depth by careful selection of patient records.

Developing Standardized Forms for Psychiatric Evaluation Data

In the past several years significant advances have been made in the translation and reduction of information on mental status and psychiatric history to a series of standardized forms applicable to psychiatric facilities. Much of this work cites only two major precedents, namely those of Pinel [1] and Adolf Meyer.[2] Pinel first detailed the recording of behavior thought to be mentally disordered, while Meyer subsequently codified a system for recording mental status that has been used up to the present time.[3-7] The recording, for each patient, of the massive amount of information suggested by Meyer in order to illustrate the patient's stream of mental activity has frequently been beyond the competence or availability of time of many clinicians. The result has been records of variable quality and depth.

In order to overcome this problem, various standardized forms have been developed. Space precludes mentioning more than a few examples. One series of forms by Beckett et al.[8] follows the psychiatric history and mental status examination as suggested by Meyer [2] and Noyes and Kolb.[9] The lists of scales of five-point and dichotomous items are summarized under the following headings: (1) identification, (2) history of present illness, (3) precipitating stress, (4) symptoms of present illness, (5) past history, (6) personal and social characteristics, (7) environment during rearing, (8) developmental history, (9) sexual history, (10) marital history, (11) history of children, (12) history of parents, (13) history of siblings, (14) mental status examination, (15) course and prognosis, and (16) 1-, 3-, and 5-year follow-up. Specialized psychiatric recording forms have been designed for use with mental hospital inpatients [10] for outpatient settings [11] and for psychiatric consultation services.[12]

Alternative methods of obtaining standardized mental status information from retrospective psychiatric records are also under investigation and show considerable promise. Once such study [13] investigated the extent to which routine psychiatric reports, more specifically admission summaries, could duplicate and be used for research purposes in place of in vivo interviews with psychiatric patients. The 20 scales which are part of the Symptom Rating Scale introduced by Jenkins, Stauffacher and Hester [14] were used to specify the information, in terms of which the reliability and validity of obtaining data from case records were measured. The findings indicated the feasibility of duplicating from records psychiatric information obtained from face to face interviews.

Another study [15], under the auspices of the Social Security Administration, was faced with the problem of having to make disability decisions regarding claimants on the basis of documentary evidence alone—a problem typical among disability insurance programs. A psychiatric review form (PRF) was developed and refined to assist in the assessment of psychiatric impairment. The final form of the inventory consisted of one page and covered the following major areas: effective intelligence, affective status, reality contact and socially deviant behaviors. Studies of the applicability and reliability of the PRF have demonstrated a high degree of acceptance and interrater agreement.

Restructured Forms of the Medical Record

A major development in the structure of the medical record has occurred with the introduction in 1968 by Weed, of problem-oriented recording. [16, 17] The principal objective is to focus attention and clinical transcription of information on the specific problems presented by the patient. These problems may either be amenable to treatment within the facility contacted, may require outside consultation, or may be referred elsewhere for treatment. Of demonstrable importance to psychiatry is that these "problems" need not represent clinical diagnostic entities or even psychiatric symptoms. Rather, they can represent any disturbance to the patient's well-being including economic difficulties, disturbances in relations within the family, serious problems in urban living or any physical or psychosomatic disorder. Their underlying assumption is that it may be fruitless to attempt to deal directly with a specific medical problem without dealing with the physical or social environment which may either influence the course of the illness itself or hinder the process of therapy.

What is suggested here is a reconceptualization of the purposes of medical recording and perhaps of the treatment process. It is not sufficient that the array of patient problems be recorded. The problem-oriented scheme requires that each problem be systematically followed up until some resolution occurs, either through the treating facility itself or by reference to outside sources. Within this framework all participating staff members are to record aspects of diagnosis, treatment and progress in relation to each problem. Thus, there are longer compartmentalized areas in the record for separate recording of physicians' notes, nursing notes, social work notes, etc. There are also remarks by individual staff members, regardless of specialty or training, who have been dealing with a specific problem.

The problem-oriented system is well suited to standardization, and even to automation and computer processing. With a specification of the types (e.g., medical, psychiatric, social, physical environmental) and subdivisions of problems that appear with some frequency, a checkoff list and categorized design of test questions can be used to translate the record into a series of standardized forms.

An important feature of the problem-oriented system is its indexing scheme in which a specification of each problem is numbered and the progress of its resolution is displayed. The sequence of treatment for any problem is then presented in the record according to its index problem number. A problem number is not dropped when a problem has been completely resolved, and therefore the sequence of problem numbers does not change. It is obvious that the complete display of all aspects of treatment as they relate to progress in each problem area is useful in utilization review. It makes possible the rapid location of information for each of a patient's problems; it furnishes evidence on the extent to which patients' problems have actually been dealt with; and it allows observation of the contribution of each staff member to each aspect of patient care. In fact, it theoretically allows such detailed scrutiny of the clinical care process that it has extraordinary utility as a teaching, evaluative and research instrument.

This problem-oriented system has gained a substantial following among health professionals in general medicine [18] and is now being further developed for use in psychiatry [19, 20]. Two excellent examples of the adaptation of the problem-oriented system in psychiatry have recently been published [21, 22]. It is clear from these examples that substantial variety will be found in such adaptations which are of necessity peculiar to the organization of care in each institution. A noteworthy difference between the two cited examples is in the manner by which estimate is made of patients' problems. In the adaptation described by Ryback and Gardner,[21] each clinician may describe different problems according to specialty and training, or even develop entirely different problem lists. In the scheme described by Novello [22], the full therapeutic team decides on a common problem list after a conference. The two schemes have the remainder of the common structure of the problem-oriented scheme in common.

The Development of Scales for the Measurement of Mental Status

Another major effort in standardization concerns the development of scales to measure mental status.[23, 24] While there is no overall agreement as to distinctive and easily identifiable measures of mental illness and specific diagnoses, it appears that the areas of major disagreement are being narrowed down by the use of comparative empirical tests among different groups of researchers [25-27] and across countries.[28] In these tests, clustering methods (especially factor analyses) are frequently used in order to reduce large pools of information on patients to a relatively small group of psychiatric syndromes, (each of which may then be indicated by answers to a selected number of objective questions). Outstanding examples are the Mental Status Schedule [29] and the Psychiatric Status Schedule [30] developed by Spitzer et al. The former is designed for use during a psychiatric interview and reports on a variety of symptoms involving intellectual and emotional disorders, impairments in role functioning, the conduct of leisure time activities and daily routine. Similarly, the Psychiatric Evaluation Form of Endicott, Spitzer et al.[31] is a rating scale designed to record scaled judgments of a subject's mental and social functioning during a one-week period.

Also widely used is another scale, the Inpatient Multidimensional Scale by Lorr and Klett [32], for the evaluation of psychotic syndromes following an interview with the patient. These syndromes have been established by repeated factor analyses based on psychotic population samples in the United States and other countries [33-35] and have a distinctive relationship to psychiatric diagnosis.[32] A final example is the SCL-90, an outpatient psychiatric rating scale developed by Derogatis et al.[11] It is a self-report clinical rating scale oriented toward the symptomatic behavior of psychiatric outpatients. This scale is comprised of 90 items which reflect nine primary symptom dimensions believed to underlie the majority of symptom behaviors observed in outpatients: (1) somatization, (2) obsessive-compulsive, (3) interpersonal sensitivity, (4) depression, (5) anxiety, (6) hostility, (7) phobic anxiety, (8) paranoid ideation and (9) psychoticism.

Automated Processing of Psychiatric Data

It is evident that the use of computerized data processing has now come into prominence in psychiatric institutions [36-39] as it previously did in general hospitals throughout the United States [40-42] and in industrial medicine.[43-46] The computer has been useful in psychiatric facilities not only as a device to aid in accounting and payrolls, but in the actual management of patient care. The use of the computer printout to indicate utilization patterns and patient flow has occurred among many institutions and in psychiatric registers.[47–50] Perhaps the most far reaching development in computer use in psychiatry has been as an aid to diagnosis and subsequent treatment.[51–54]

As a diagnostic aid the computer serves in much the same way as multiphasic screening. The objective is to jog the clinician's memory so that a certain standard group of signs and symptoms is investigated for all patients regardless of their presenting problems. The group of theoretically possible signs and symptoms is presented to the clinician on a standardized form of the type discussed earlier in this chapter. A series of checkoff lists, multiple-choice items, scales of presence or severity of specific signs or symptoms, in addition to other standardized measures, is then responded to by the clinician. Standardized diagnoses or symptom clusters may then become the basis of the clinical statement of the patient's problem. Similarly, the variety of treatment alternatives is represented on protocol forms, and the clinician indicates his choice.

While automated data systems in psychiatric care are certainly not necessary to the process of utilization review, they are quite useful. Computerization of psychiatric information not only allows vast amounts of data on patients to be permanently stored and rapidly retrieved, but also permits rapid sorting of all stored data and display of the sorted information in easily read tabulations. The procedural ease of this sorting process also allows access to critical details in each patient record stored within the system. Thus, regardless of the criterion by which a utilization review committee may be selecting charts for review (diagnosis, specific problem such as suicide, age, sex, "randomness," etc.) the computer will produce a file of patient charts for review based on one or several simultaneous criteria.

DEVELOPMENT OF A STANDARDIZED RECORDING SYSTEM

The existence of a standardized recording system is central to the mechanics of utilization review. Therefore, the first task of the PURE research group concerned with data gathering and analysis was to assure the presence of an adequate base of information. The information system to be designed and constructed at the Connecticut Mental Health Center for use by PURE was ideally to incorporate the following specifications:

1. It was to include a sufficiently large sample so as to enable efficient utilization review,
2. The type and number of variables involved were to cover as many topics as are pertinent to utilization review,
3. The sample was to cover a sufficient period of time so as to enable reasonably accurate estimates of changes in patterns of patient care over time.

Estimates of Quality of Clinical Records

Abstracting of the clinical record in current use was the principal method of constructing the data base. Thus, the means by which the feasibility of developing such an information system was estimated relied largely on: (1) the adequacy of data then found in the clinical records and (2) the skill of the coding (or abstracting) staff in accurately drawing a large number of data from the records.

In order to obtain an estimate of the accuracy of clinical records, a 20 percent sample of all charts for 1968–69 admissions to CMHC was checked for the treatment plan. Errors were found in five percent of these charts, which indicates that overall the data on file were of relatively high quality. The discharge date accounted for approximately 62 percent of all errors found, and rarely was more than one error found in any one record.

During the second year of the study, the sociodemographic data and much of utilization of service data were obtained through precoded MSIS forms rather than hand-coded via abstracted forms. As a result the errors were reduced from five percent to two percent. Thus there are only minimal difficulties in securing accurate information by abstracting psychiatric data for purposes of utilization review. The most common problems in coding from the chart record to the coded form were: (1) handwritten material was sometimes illegible, (2) the clinician was not explicit, (3) diagnoses were hard to locate or entirely missing, (4) it was difficult to determine whether a patient was discharged, (5) there was no evidence of the physician's decision or signature to administer drugs, even though there were abundant indications that drugs had been dispensed, and (6) there were periods when substantial numbers of charts were out to clinicians on the service. Besides being a nuisance, obtaining a chart which had been aimlessly lying on a desk for many weeks was very time consuming. Besides establishing the accuracy of the records, the coding supervisor checked for reliability by having the six coders abstract the same fifteen charts without being aware of this duplication. The results showed an overall error of three percent. Thus there was a high level of reliability as well as validity in the abstracting system.

Interrelationships among Data Systems

An important stage in the development of psychiatric information systems involves the merger of data from different sources, especially from different institutions. This is of particular importance in psychiatric utilization review, which frequently employs clinical norms as standards for care. Thus the larger the patient population covered by a particular norm or clinical practice, the more reliable will be the statistical comparability of actual practice. A relatively large patient population whose care is under examination, across institutions or regions, is also important in the construction of more universally valid and pertinent norms for case management.

The existence of standardized information systems, perhaps based on similar facilities (e.g., inpatient, outpatient, community mental health center, general hospital) or regions (especially on a statewide basis) has recently begun to form the basis for comparative analyses. The PURE Project itself utilized the Multi-State Information System (MSIS), housed at the Rockland State Hospital in Orangeburg, New York, as the basis for its comparative studies of mental health center utilization in four states. The institutions involved were the Connecticut Mental Health Center (New Haven, Connecticut), the Erich Lindemann Mental Health Center (Boston), the Rockland State Hospital Mental Health Center (Orangeburg, New York) and the Area B Mental Health Center (Washington, D.C.).

The Multi-State Information System for Psychiatric Patients (MSIS) is a comprehensive, computer-based system designed to provide both automated clinical information and a management support system for patients in participating psychiatric facilities. Currently, Connecticut, Hawaii, Massachusetts, New York, Rhode Island, Vermont and the District of Columbia are participating either via terminals linked to the computer at Rockland State Hospital, by mail or on state-owned, independent computers.

The system is designed to follow the patient through all phases of psychiatric service, whether the patient is being treated in an inpatient facility or in other psychiatric settings such as clinics and community mental health centers. Usually, information about a patient is recorded on preprinted questionnaires de-signed to record those data normally gathered in the treatment process. The admission form provides the basic data needed to open a file. It establishes the identity of the patient, records the initial ward/unit assignment and enters basic demographic data, an appraisal of presenting problems, information about pre-vious psychiatric service and source of referral. Once the patient's file is on record, the full gamut of services rendered by psychiatric facilities—ranging from brief, non-clinical contacts to the long-term treatment of chronically ill patients—can be captured on MSIS forms.

The forms are generally multiple-choice check lists; the person com-pleting the form need choose only those items appropriate for the individual patient. Moreover, the forms are designed as an integrated group, so that the same data need not be repeatedly collected. For example, once diagnosis on admission is marked on the admission form and stored in the data base, it is retrieved each time the initial diagnosis is needed for a report.

Although current MSIS forms are general in their application, addi-tional forms are being designed to capture special kinds of information. For example, an abbreviated, combination admission/termination form to be used for single visit cases such as those encountered in emergency rooms is being planned. Admission and termination forms as well as a mental status examination form specifically geared to children are other examples of specialized forms being designed.

Once data have been recorded as part of the clinical process, they are either sent by mail or transmitted over telephone lines from terminals located in facilities in each cooperating state to the central computer. Clinical, administrative and research reports are later transmitted from the computer center and printed at the appropriate terminal.

The merger of the data system of the Connecticut Mental Health Center with that of MSIS required a greater effort then was anticipated initially. The problems inherent in the merger of these systems are probably typical for the interdigitation of psychiatric or medical information systems in general. In the case of the PURE Project, it was possible to document those problems and the progress in finding solutions.

Characteristics of the Merged Information System

The data system included patient information based upon two years of admissions to and contacts with the CMHC during 1968–69 and 1969–70. (The 1968–69 data contain 48 variables on a population of 1849 persons, while the 1969–70 data contain 158 separate variables on a population of 3649 patients.) Our use of several of the MSIS precoded forms was instrumental in our ability to derive over 100 additional variables for the second year's sample. During the first year nearly all of the data obtained were gleaned from the psychiatric records on the basis of a coded set of abstracts. Many of the second year's data, by contrast, were obtained through precoded forms which were part of the psychiatric record —either MSIS or CMHC developed forms. In addition to the basic two-year sample, a 20 percent sample of admissions to CMHC during 1969–70 was obtained for purposes of abstracting pertinent information relative to detailed treatment plan and actual course of treatment.(See Appendix 3-A) Overall, the following classes of data were obtained for the sample years:

1. Sociodemographic variables
2. Previous treatment (if any)
3. Diagnostic information on admission and discharge
4. Source of referral to CMHC and point of referral from CMHC
5. Unit of treatment
6. Type, frequency and duration of specific treatment
7. Type of drug
8. Mode of determination of treatment

In addition, for 1969–70, estimates of mental status and an estimate of the extent of improvement in the patient's condition at discharge, based on MSIS forms, were included.

INITIAL MERGER OF THE INFORMATION
SYSTEMS, 1969–70

Two central problems surrounded the merger of the two information systems: (1) the multipurpose character of the storage and retrieval systems and (2)

Data Group
Treatment Plan Variables

INSTRUCTIONS

1. Definitions of terms:

   Unit = a distinct outpatient, inpatient, or day hospital service.

   Episode = a continuous enrollment in a specific unit, unbroken by any lengthy period of non-attendance.

   Treatment Plan = a specific statement by a clinician, usually made at the time of Admission to a unit and included in an Admission Summary or on p. 10 of the Patient Abstract.

   Treatment = a specific form of care, therapy, or medication. There are usually several different treatments for each episode.

2. Definitions of treatment:

   Individual therapy = where a patient is seen by a clinician alone. Short term therapy is usually less than two months in length.

   Group therapy = where a patient meets with other patients under the supervision of a clinician.

   Family therapy = consultation involving members of a patient's family or actually where members of the family are taken into therapy.

3. Non-overnight Emergency Room visits: these should not be included in the coding. In other words, disregard all yellow ER forms, unless they denote an overnight stay on the ETU unit.

4. A new card should be filled out:
   a. every time a unit is changed
   b. every time a clinician is changed
   c. every time there is a significant gap in time between treatments
   d. every time a new Treatment Plan is introduced

5. There is room for three different treatments (in Actual Course of Treatment)

on each card. If there are more than three treatments for one episode (i.e.,
Group Therapy, Individual Therapy, Family Therapy, and Librium medication), fill out a new card with the additional treatments. Number the card
(variable 3, column 3) two, etc., fill in columns 1, 2, 3, 4, 5, 6, and 7 the same
as the first card, and skip from 8 to 25. In space 25–26 of the second card
begin to record all treatments in excess of three. (Disregard cols. 66–69
on second card).

Definitions of Treatments (for Variable 6 of Code Structure)

00 = no treatment indicated.

01 = evaluation only.

(used when a patient is seen only once or twice for evaluation for other treatment; otherwise, *evaluation* should not be listed as a separate treatment. The assumption is that evaluation and the first treatment therapy are combined).

02 = individual OP therapy, unspecified time.

(used primarily with Treatment Plan instead of Actual Course of Treatment; indicates that the patient and the doctor meet on a one-to-one basis, but no information is present concerning the nature of the admission).

03 = individual OP therapy, short term.

(same Rx as above, but for less than two months. Used to describe follow-up OP service and brief treatment during periods of crisis).

04 = individual OP therapy, long term.

(same Rx as above, but for longer than two months).

05 = individual IP therapy, with doctor.

(same Rx as above, but usually on a more frequent basis, while patient is an inpatient).

06 = individual IP therapy, with Nurse, Psy. Aide, or MSW.

(same Rx as above, but without a doctor present; this includes the general category of *patient-staff* meetings also, even though the patient is not alone in these circumstances).

07 = individual OP therapy,
Nurse, Psy. Aide, or
MSW.

(same Rx as above, but with a clinician
other than a doctor; usually found exclusively in follow-up cases).

08 = group OP therapy,
unspecified time.

(treatment involving a clinician, the
patient, and other individuals, who are
not defined).

09 = group OP therapy,
short term.

(same Rx as above, but less than two
months in duration and usually centering
around a crisis situation).

10 = group OP therapy,
long term.

(same Rx as above, but for a period
longer than two months).

11 = group OP couples
therapy.

(treatment involving the patient, his or
her spouse, and other married couples;
no time length need be indicated).

12 = group IP therapy,
unspecified type.

(treatment involving a patient and an
undefined group; this SHOULD *NOT*
include Inpatient Community Meetings.
Community Meetings and Milieu Therapy
involve all inpatients; hence they are not
considered as distinct Rx).

13 = group IP conjoint
therapy.

(treatment involving a patient, members of his family in some cases, and
more than one clinician).

14 = group IP collateral
therapy.

(treatment in which the patient is seen
by one clinician and a member or members of his family are seen by another
clinician at another time).

15 = individual family
therapy.

(treatment involving the patient, his
family, and *one* clinician).

16 = multi-family therapy.

(treatment involving several patients
and their families, plus a clinician).

17 = family therapy OP,
    unspecified type.

(treatment involving a patient and his family, but with no further qualification mentioned).

18 = family involvement.

(a service in which members of a patient's family or friends are interviewed, as opposed to being incorporated into Rx, by a Clinician . . . but rarely a doctor; this category should be used unless the Treatment Plan specifies *collateral therapy*, since the latter implies concurrent patient involvement).

19 = family therapy IP,
    unspecified type.

(treatment involving a patient and his family, but with no further qualification mentioned).

20 = inpatient service,
    unspecified treatment,
    short term.

(a general category to be used when no specific treatments are mentioned for an inpatient; short term applies to all ETU inpatients and to others who are seen on a crisis basis in HWH, GCD, or Research; two weeks is usually the dividing line between short and long term).*

21 = inpatient service,
    unspecified treatment,
    long term.

(same Rx as above, but for periods longer than two weeks).*

22 = vocational and Edu-
    cational rehabilitation.

(rehabilitation therapy undertaken at CMHC or referred from CMHC while patient is still active).

23 = waiting list.

(designates a period in which the patient, who has been evaluated, is waiting for specific OP treatment).

---

*These two treatment classifications should be used primarily to describe Treatment Plans where no mention is made of precise Rx, like individual or group therapy. When using either #21 or #20 with Actual Course of Treatment, there should be no other treatment information available, with the exception of drug data.

24 = same treatment as before, but new clinician.

(used solely with Treatment Plan to indicate that a patient has changed doctors, but not treatment; this usually occurs during the July rotation when new residents come to the hospital).

25 = group couples IP therapy, with MSW or Psyc. Aide.

(same Rx as #11, but without a doctor).

26 = evaluation for outside CMHC.

(evaluation in which CMHC doctor is performing a service for another facility with prior knowledge that the patient will not be taken into therapy at CMHC).

27 = group therapy DH, unspecified type.

(same Rx as #08, but for Day Hospital).

28 = patient refused Rx.

(used in Actual Course of Treatment to indicate that a treatment was recommended, but not undertaken).

29 = after-care group.

(unspecified group therapy directed by the CMHC in which a discharged patient is involved on an informal basis).

30 through 70 . . . . . these are specific medication categories which are self-explanatory . . . .

97 = phone contact.

(this category pertains to a post-evaluation service in which the patient is not critical enough to warrant regular OP care; phone contact between the clinician and the patient is maintained).

98 = field worker visits, concurrent with regular treatment.

(where a field worker visits the home of a regular OP patient).

99 = neurological consultation.

(treatment of a diagnostic type undertaken at YNHH, usually by Dr. Mattson, at the behest of a CMHC clinician).

TREATMENT PLAN

Variable	Columns	Description
1	1	Number of this admission 1 = first admission 2 = second admission, etc.
2	2	Number of this episode 1 = first episode of a given admission 2 = second episode, etc.
3	3	Number of the card for particular episode 1 = first card for a particular episode 2 = second card (where applicable)
4	4–7	Patient I-D Number, last 4 digits
5	8–9	*Unit Assigned in Treatment Plan* 10 = GCD DH 11 = GCD IP 12 = GCD ETU 13 = HWH IP 14 = HWH DH 15 = HWH OP 16 = Research IP 18 = GCD OP 19 = Drug Dependency 20 = Depression Study 21 = ECOP 26 = ETU Follow-up 27 = Research OP 28 = Research DH 33 = Field Service

(all units below came into operation after July 1, 1969)
32 = EBT (HWH) + Evaluation
33 = HWH Medication and Socialization
34 = GCD EBT + Evaluation
35 = PCL

Treatment Recommended in Treatment Plan

Variable	Columns	Description
6	10–11	00 = no treatment indicated 01 = evaluation only 02 = individual OP therapy (unspec. time) 03 = individual OP therapy (short term)

04 = individual OP therapy (long term)
05 = individual IP therapy (with clinician)
06 = individual IP therapy (with MSW or nurse, P.A.)
07 = individual OP therapy (Patient-Staff Meetings)
08 = group OP therapy (unspec. time)
09 = group OP therapy (short term)
10 = group OP therapy (long term)
11 = group OP couples therapy
12 = group IP therapy (unspec.)
13 = group IP conjoint therapy (Family)
14 = group IP collateral therapy (Family)
15 = individual Family therapy (pt. present)
16 = multi-family therapy
17 = family therapy (unspec. type) OP
18 = family involvement (family or friends'
         interviews)
19 = family therapy (unspec. type) IP
20 = Inpatient service, unspecified treatment,
         short term (ETU)
21 = Inpatient service, unspecified treatment,
         long term
22 = Vocational and Educational Rehabilitation
23 = Waiting List
24 = Same Treatment as before, but new clinician
25 = Group Couples inpatient therapy (with SW)
26 = Evaluation for referral outside of CMHC
27 = Group Day Hospital therapy (unspec.)
28 = Patient refused treatment
29 = After-care group
80 = Unit refused to accept patient into Rx
87 = Staff Status (IP) (Post Aug. 1968)
88 = Community status (IP) (Post Aug. 1968)
89 = Family Status (IP) (Post Aug. 1968)
93 = Outpatient Addicts Subcommittee
94 = DH (unspec. Rx)
95 = OP couples Group with MSW or Psyc. Aide
96 = ETU Day Status
97 = Phone Contact
98 = Concurrent Field Worker visits to Patient's
         Home
99 = Neurological Consultation (YNHH)

30 = Medication maintenance (unspecified drug)	41 = Mellaril	53 = Valium
	42 = Methadone	54 = Coumadin

31 = Benadryl
32 = Cogentin
33 = Colace
34 = Compazine
35 = Darvon
36 = Elavil
37 = Haldol
38 = Kemadrin
39 = Librium
40 = Lithium

43 = Noludar
44 = Potassium Triplex
45 = Prolixin
46 = Seconal
47 = Stelazine
48 = Thorazine
49 = Tiractin
50 = Tofranil
51 = Trilafon
52 = Trilafon & Congentin

55 = ECT
56 = Ritalin
57 = Dilantin
58 = Deprol
59 = Norflex
60 = Sustogen
61 = Digoxin
62 = Vivactin

Variable	Columns	Description
7	12–13	Treatment recommended No. 2
8	14–15	Treatment recommended No. 3
9	16–17	Treatment recommended No. 4
10	18–19	Treatment recommended No. 5
11	20–21	Treatment recommended No. 6
12	22–23	Length of time for proposed treatment:

00 = DATA NOT AVAILABLE
01 = one visit
02 = less than one week
03 = between one week and two weeks
04 = one month or less
05 = three months or less
06 = six months or less
07 = nine months or less
08 = one year or less
09 = more than one year
10 = as long as necessary
11 = until the July rotation

13	24	Pattern of proposed treatments:

1 = one visit or extended evaluation
2 = day-to-day treatment (i.e., DH or ETU follow-up); also includes day-to-day drug maintenance
3 = one visit per week
4 = more than one visit per week
5 = one visit per month or more
6 = as needed; PRN; less than one visit per month
7 = border status (IP)
8 = not applicable (waiting list)

9 = infrequent or sporadic attendance; no
regular pattern; infrequent drug
maintenance
0 = DATA NOT AVAILABLE

ACTUAL COURSE OF TREATMENT

Variable	*Columns*	*Description*
14	25-26	Unit actually assigned (Use CODE for Variable 5)
	27-28	First Type of Treatment (Use CODE for Variable 6)
	29-33	Date Treatment was begun (month, day, and last digit of year)
	34-38	Date Treatment was ended (Last completed visit to OP)
	39	Pattern of Treatment (Use CODE for Variable 13)
15	40-41	Second Type of Treatment
	42-43	Date begun
	47-51	Date ended
	52	Pattern
16	53-54	Third Type of Treatment
	55-59	Date Begun
	60-64	Date Ended
	65	Pattern

N.B. If there are more than three treatments for a single episode, make out a
second card, fill in columns 1, 2, 4-7 the same as the first card; place a 2 (or 3,
etc. depending on number of treatments) in column 3; skip columns 8-24; begin
coding in column 25. Disregard columns 66-69 on second card.

Chapter Four

Epidemiologic and Ecologic Analyses

Jerzy E. Henisz
Gary L. Tischler
Jerome K. Myers

Ecologic and epidemiologic studies have a substantive role in both patient care and evaluation and utilization review. By facilitating a systematic inquiry into the extent and character of the interaction between a mental health service program and the population being served, such studies can be used as sensitive indicators of provider performance. The data supply information related to the characteristics of a population at risk (potential consumers of service) and the characteristics of those currently being served by existing agencies (the actual consumers of service). In the pages to follow, we shall sketch a basic approach for the systematic use of this information, both to evaluate help-seeking behaviors, service utilization patterns and the availability and accessibility of care and to clarify issues related to the need versus the demand for service.

THE MEASUREMENT OF NEED

To gain some estimate of the need for service in a particular area, it is necessary to study the prevalence of treated, untreated or even unrecognized disorder within the community, as well as a cluster of factors associated with the emergence of symptoms, subjective perceptions of individual health needs and the willingness to accept psychiatric care, and the availability of service in terms of place, time, quality and cost. A mental health survey provides the most accurate information of this type. If such a method is used, however, attention must be paid to insuring (1) good sampling procedure, (2) a well prepared and pretested interview schedule, and (3) well trained interviewers who know the neighborhood being surveyed and are not perceived as intruders.

Mental Health Surveys

In survey research, the approach to sample selection is crucial if the statistical validity of the conclusions is to be insured. Information obtained through interviews, and figures calculated on the basis of aggregate data are representative of the population only insofar as each member of the community under study has an equal chance to be included in a survey. Ideally, sample selections should be on the basis of full census data. Subjects for the representative sample should be identified either through the use of tables of random numbers or by computer. When full census data are not available or access to them is barred, a variety of other lists can be substituted (e.g., telephone books, voting lists, local addresses). To the degree that these lists do not cover an entire population, however, the representativeness of the sample will be jeopardized. An alternative sampling method allows one to select households randomly (first step) and then individuals living in those households (second step). The exact proportion of the total population included in the representative sample is usually determined by a statistician. It is a rule of thumb that samples significantly smaller than 1000 are useless for epidemiological estimates of psychiatric disorder. A sample much larger than 1000 is rarely needed unless the study is nationwide.

The interview schedule should provide information about the sample in a standardized way to insure that each individual is asked more or less the same questions within the same context. A typical interview schedule garners basic sociodemographic data about both the respondent and the respondent's family and focuses upon questions related to social and geographical mobility, role performance, life events in a defined period of time, expectations for future changes, familiarity with and utilization of existing social, health and psychiatric faculties, physical and emotional disorders experienced in the past, symptoms associated with emotional distress, and willingness to seek and accept help when experiencing such symptoms. A number of inventories and scales used for assessing mental status in the field survey situation have been described in the literature.[1-10]

The selection and training of skillful interviewers is of great importance for insuring that potential subjects are reached. According to Cochran, "a return of above or about 90 percent of the selected sample should be aimed for and is feasible." To assure so high a rate of return, interviewers must be carefully screened and briefed about the nature of the project. They must be prepared to work evenings and weekends to accommodate respondents and should demonstrate good familiarity with the interview schedule before entering the field. In some cases it is advisable to have interviewers who speak foreign languages and translate the interview schedule into whatever languages reflect the ethnic background of the community.

The Mental Health Demographic Profile System

An alternative model for estimating mental health needs involves the use of census socioeconomic data. It is a correlative model built upon the assumption that certain population characteristics predict high risk in terms of the need for mental health and other social and health services. The model makes use of data that are less focused and comprehensive than those obtained through a mental health survey. It does not permit an accurate approximation of the prevalence of mental disorder in the community of personal factors influencing the perception of need or the translation of that perception into help-seeking behaviors. Despite these limitations, for a given program, it represents a less costly and time consuming approach for estimating the need for mental health service.

NIMH has taken the leadership in developing this model. [12, 13] A data source is now available for each community mental health catchment area in the United States as well as for each census tract, county and state. The system includes information on the distribution of the population by age, sex, color and marital status. Profiles have also been constructed on the basis of specific social and economic variable from the 1970 census that contain extensive data on six broad social areas: socioeconomic status, ethnic composition, household composition and family structure, style of life, condition of housing, and community instability.

THE EXPRESSED DEMAND FOR SERVICE

Mental health survey results may vary according to the location of the study and to the specific operational definition of psychological impairment. Since 1950, however, most field studies suggest that between fifteen and twenty percent of the population exhibit high symptomatology. The proportion of mildly disturbed may run as high as 80 percent. Translating these figures into meaningful data for planning and developing mental health services, however, requires close scrutiny of the other end of the "need-demand continuum"—the expressed demand for services reflected by admissions to extant mental health facilities.

In counting admissions to mental health facilities it is important to begin by defining what represents a case. Generally, the definition is operationalized to include all individuals who either come or are brought to a mental health facility for care. This definition focuses upon a behavioral end-point that is measurable and does not take into account whether there is evidence of an illness condition. To avoid overcounting, one has to assume that the request for care is for the applicant, an approach which creates some confusion if a spouse requests help because of marital discord or a family member seeks help because of problems in the family. The couple or family may end up utilizing one unit of service (e.g., one hour of family counseling) but be registered as two or five "cases."

The dilemma of case definition is further confounded by differing institutional practices. To "come" or "be brought" may or may not include telephone contacts ("May I see somebody?" "Yes. Please give me some information about yourself. We have walk-in service. Come down immediately.") or preadmission screening ("Given the nature of your problem, I think that your needs would be best met if you contacted family service. It isn't necessary for you to be admitted here.") One must, therefore, know the institutions and their admission policies in order to avoid producing confusing, misleading and totally uncomparable data.

In addition to case definition, the definition of a mental health facility may also present the investigator studying expressed demand some difficulties. State hospitals, mental health centers, inpatient psychiatric units, day hospitals and psychiatric clinics will, of course, be placed on the list. Correctional institutions employing mental health professionals, facilities for mental retardates, halfway houses or nursing homes for discharged psychiatric patients, however, may or may not be included. Family counseling services, sex clinics, parental guidance clinics and other facilities providing many services identical to those offered by mental health institutions are often not included since they eschew membership in a formal mental health service matrix and prefer to dissociate themselves from any effort that may even symbolically link them with such organizations.

The data on cases admitted to mental health facilities are frequently displayed in terms of new- and re-admission rates per one, ten or hundred thousand of either the general population or age-, sex-, and race-specific subgroups within the general population. Here again, some caution must be exercised. The rates may be misleading epidemiologically not only because of the reasons previously mentioned but also because of duplicated counts resulting from a single individual having multiple admissions, during the same year, to a single institution or to different institutions.

As these examples suggest, an adequate description of expressed demand may prove as difficult a task as investigating the need for service through a mental health survey. The unavailability of data related to service utilization may lead to a situation where the enormity of the gap between demand and need may, to a certain extent, be a product of the overestimation of need and the underestimation of actual demand. Although the information on expressed demand may be considered misleading by an epidemiologist interested in getting hard data, they serve useful purposes in describing trends in the actual demand and consumption of services.

Two Studies of Expressed Demand

A federally funded community mental health center has the responsibility to provide or arrange mental health care for all residents of a defined geographical area. To test one center's success in achieving this objective, a comparative study was undertaken of admissions to four agencies to which residents of a particular catchment had access. The agencies included a mental health center (MHC), a state hospital (SH), a private psychiatric clinic (PPC) and a general hospital emergency room (ER). The ER and MHC are affiliated programs, 24-hour emergency coverage being provided at the general hospital. One year's admission rates per 1000 eligible residents were calculated from data abstracted from agency case records.

As table 4-1 indicates, ER and MHC provide the bulk of psychiatric services. PPC furnishes only a small amount of care. While the clinic's fee schedule may act as a potential utilization barrier, the results suggest that the existence of the MHC does not deprive citizens of the option of seeking services from a private facility. It should also be noted that for every two catchment residents admitted to MHC, one was sent to the state hospital. This relatively high admission figure to the state hospital stimulated further inquiry into the question of equity of service as a function of race and age.

The data presented in table 4-2 demonstrates similar race-related admission patterns for all agencies except PPC. Non-whites are admitted at rates approximately twice those of whites. Age specific comparisons, however, yield different results (see table 4-3). While ER and PPC do not show any specific pattern in terms of their clients age distribution, state hospital admissions are overrepresented in all age groups above 34 and MHC admissions from the catchment are overrepresented in the age groups between 15 and 24. Thus, young people from the catchment are more likely to receive treatment from the mental health center whereas middle aged and older individuals are likely to be admitted to the state hospital.

Limiting studies of expressed demand solely to the mental health service network, however, may produce misleading findings. Under certain circumstances one might find a reduction in the demand for mental health services at the same time that the welfare, corrections, or general health systems report major increases in admissions. An ecologic perspective assumes systems interaction (i.e., each system produces output which may then become a part of input to another system). At the level of an individual client, for example, the psychiatric sector makes a statement about a client's disability, welfare supports the patient or his family, the police cope with occasional turmoil and threats to others, circuit or family courts attempt to deal with the outcome of arguments, and the juvenile court gets referrals of youngsters raised in a pathogenic environment. While not all inclusive, this example suggests that the incidents, referrals or problems dealt with by these diverse systems may well be interrelated if not identical.

To explore this issue in greater detail, the data matrix used in the

Table 4-1. Admission Rates from a Catchment Area to Four Service Agencies over a One-Year Period (rate/1000).

Emergency Room	State Hospital	Private Psychiatric Clinic	Mental Health Center
11.7	6.2	1.2	13.0

Table 4-2.   Admission Rates from Suburban and Inner-City Sections of a Catchment Area to Four Service Agencies as a Function of Race (rates/1000).[a]

	Mental Health Center	Emergency Room	State Hospital	Private Psychiatric Clinic
Inner City				
White	14.8	15.0	8.1	2.5
Non-white	29.9	37.6	20.2	1.5
Suburban				
White	5.0	5.0	3.3	.9
Non-white	8.0	8.0	5.9	.0

[a]The catchment is separated into inner city and suburban components because of the differing racial composition of the two communities.

previous analysis, expanded to include one year's utilization of the Juvenile Court, Circuit Court and Emergency Squad of the Fire Department, was correlated with the utilization of mental health services. Incidents (e.g., status violations, emergency calls, treatment episodes) rather than individuals were treated as the units of information and computed for each block-group within the catchment. A profile of reported incidents, court referrals or psychiatric admissions was then developed for each block-group and formed the baseline data for the correlation analysis presented in table 4-4.

The table is illustrative of a particular model of analysis rather than a "final" result. Without replicating the study at a different time and identifying common factors related to facility use, we should use caution in interpreting the data. The relatively high intercorrelations obtained, however, underline the importance of examining the use of alternative service systems when studying the expressed demand for mental health care.

Table 4-3.   Admissions from a Catchment Area to Four Service Agencies as a Function of Age (percent of admissions).

Age	Mental Health Center (N = 965)	Emergency Room (N = 871)	State Hospital (N = 459)	Private Psychiatric Clinic (N = 91)
15–17	8.2	6.4	1.9	3.2
18–19	8.7	7.6	7.6	4.3
20–24	29.4	20.0	19.3	42.8
25–34	26.7	29.1	25.4	20.8
35–44	13.3	16.5	17.2	7.6
45–54	8.8	11.7	19.8	12.0
55–64	3.0	5.8	5.2	8.7
65–74	1.6	2.5	3.2	0.0

Table 4–4. Correlation between Admissions to Psychiatric Services and Utilization of Other Institutions. (Coefficients computed for block-groups of catchment area.)

	Community Mental Health Center	Emergency Room	Private Psychiatric Clinic	Juvenile Court	Circuit Court	Fire Department
Community Mental Health Center	–					
Emergency Room	.89	–				
Private Psychiatric Clinic	.64	.59	–			
Juvenile Court	.83	.89	.62	–		
Circuit Court	.56	.70	.51	.76	–	
Fire Department	.85	.88	.73	.91	.79	–

THE INTERACTION BETWEEN NEED
AND DEMAND

There is ample evidence in the literature to suggest that symptomatology identified by a mental health survey may have been induced by stressful events in a
temporary situation and be a transient phenomenon rather than the manifestation of basic persistent psychological disorder.[14–16] Similarly, the epidemiological analysis of admissions suggests a strong dependence of help-seeking
behavior upon variables such as age, race, social class and distance to facility.
[17–19] One may assume, therefore, that mental status or symptoms of psychological distress are but two of the factors influencing why people come to a
mental health facility. It is through the study of the interaction between need
and demand, however, that one is able to isolate those factors which determine
help-seeking behaviors and service utilization patterns within the community. Up
to this point, we have focused upon the method and problems encountered in
measuring both need and demand. Let us now move to a detailed consideration
of the application of these methods in the systematic study of the need-demand
continuum.

THE USE OF CENSUS DATA TO STUDY THE
NEED-DEMAND CONTINUUM

Importance of Distance

Classic epidemiologic studies of admissions to psychiatric hospitals
demonstrate a strong inverse relationship between distance and utilization (Jar-
vis's law). To gain a better understanding of the role of distance on admission to
mental health facilities an attempt was made to assess the relative contribution of
distance and socioeconomic status together. The scale used to estimate socioeconomic status (SES) is a composite derived from census data which permitted
use of a person's address to estimate SES. The variables given weight by the
census group were (1) family income, (2) occupational status, (3) educational
attainment, (4) housing quality and (5) family organization. The block-groups in
New Haven were then ranked on each characteristic and assigned a SES rating.
[20] The approach made it possible to compare the geographic areas from which
patients came on a finer scale, calculate the distance from CMHC and evaluate
the effect of distance and SES on the utilization of services.

To assure a large number of data and the variations of distance
needed to discover meaningful associations, all admissions to a community
mental health center and psychiatric admission to the emergency room of a
general hospital in the city of New Haven were included in the analysis. After
determining the overall utilization rates, an attempt was made to assess the relative contribution of each factor (SES and distance) independently. The size of
the population in each SES within a fixed radius from the center and the hospital

is known; on this basis, the number of patients that would be expected to appear at each of these facilities can be estimated. If distance exerts no effect, then the observed number of patients will match the expected according to the social class composition of the population. The results are presented in table 4-5.

Distance is seen to exert a differential effect. SES groups 1 and 2 (high socioeconomic status) are hardly affected, while SES groups 3 and 4 show an inverse relationship with overrepresentation of lower class patients within a one mile radius and underrepresentation of those at a distance over two miles from the hospital. One of the factors which may account for the lack of perfect agreement in these trends is that radial distance was calculated and not transportation routes. The findings strongly suggest that proximity of service encourages greater utilization by residents from disadvantaged areas.[21]

The Comparative Study of Service Delivery Systems

Epidemiologic studies of mental illness in the community have led to the identification of populations at risk—individuals within the community more susceptible to symptom and behavior patterns indicative of emotional disorder. Utilization studies, conversely, have demonstrated a bias against the allocation of services in the community to certain of these populations. The bias is particularly strong for those in lower economic, social and ethnic groups—the poor, the non-white, the uneducated.

The empirical demonstration of a discrepancy between the need for care and the allocation of services was instrumental in the articulation of equity as a social-policy objective of the federal community mental health center program. Most broadly stated, the principle of equity of service assigns a designated center the responsibility for providing or arranging comprehensive, coordinated mental health care for all residents of a geographically defined catchment in need of service. Since the principle of equity applies to all catchment residents irrespective of whether they are rich or poor, black or white, acutely disturbed or chronically ill, it inherently counters extant bias in the allocation of mental health services and moves toward insuring their availability to populations at risk previously denied them.

To test the degree of success achieved by a federally funded mental health center program, we asked two major evaluative questions: Can catchmenting be shown to be associated with measurable differences in terms of who is served by a mental health program? Does the availability of catchment oriented services influence patterns in the use of mental health services? To answer these questions, a design was adopted that called for comparing the use of an emergency room and a mental health service complex by both catchmented and non-catchmented populations. The emergency room of Yale–New Haven Hospital and the Connecticut Mental Health Center provided the locus for the studies. Together these facilities offer 24-hour psychiatric care to a population of more than 300,000.

Table 4-5. Relationship between Socioeconomic Status and Distance

| | | Emergency Room Psychiatric Admissions | | | | | |
| | | 1 mile radius | | | 2+ miles radius | | |
SES	Rate/1000 New Haven Proper	Difference between Observed and Estimated Admissions[a]	z-Score	P	Difference between Observed and Estimated Admissions[a]	z-Score	P
1	7.0	+ 9.0	1.87	N.S.	−10.8	.81	N.S.
2	11.4	− 22.0	1.65	N.S.	−19.4	.83	N.S.
3	18.2	+119.8	5.65	$<.001$	−92.1	4.29	$<.001$
4	24.0	+ 48.6	1.76	N.S.	−21.2	2.38	$<.05$
		Mental Health Center Admissions					
1	10.3	− .9	.26	N.S.	− 8.5	.63	N.S.
2	12.3	− 4.0	.59	N.S.	−14.1	.83	N.S.
3	15.8	+ 97.2	4.76	$<.001$	−75.2	3.57	$<.001$
4	18.1	+ 82.5	3.13	$<.01$	−18.4	2.22	$<.05$

[a] (+) indicates observed admissions $>$ estimated; (−) indicates $<$.

At the time of the studies, the mental health center was divided into two major clinical units that shared a common facility. The general clinical division (GCD) was organized as a multiservice treatment facility. It consisted of a number of autonomous subunits, each responsible for a discrete task such as emergency treatment, outpatient care, partial hospitalization or inpatient care. Although it accepted patients from a region consisting of New Haven and twelve surrounding towns, the GCD maintained a task rather than a population orientation (figure 4-1).

The Hill-West Haven Division (HWD), on the other hand, maintained a strong catchment orientation. Funded under the Community Mental Health Centers Act of 1963, the division offered a range of adult clinical services comparable to the GCD but limited to a geographically defined area that included an inner city neighborhood of some 21,000 and a working class suburb of 54,000. These services were structured to maximize continuity of care through the use of team mechanisms linking the division's intramural and outreach programs.

The research plan called for comparing the ER-GCD with the ER-HWH patient population to determine the extent to which the concept of geographic responsibility was associated with observable differences in the utilization of mental health services by both high-risk groups and the general population. A straightforward comparison would have been misleading or uninterpretable, however, because of differences in total size, geographical distribution and socioeconomic characteristics of the base population from which the patients were

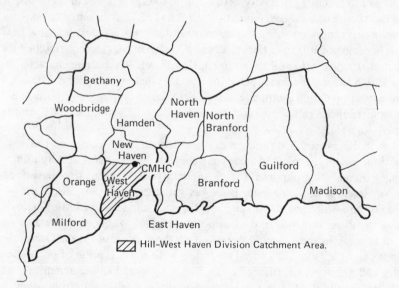

Figure 4-1. Connecticut Mental Health Center Primary Service Region

drawn. Controls, therefore, had to be introduced to insure homogeneity within and between the two populations being studied. Put another way, it was necessary to create a "dummy catchment" from which the multitreatment facility would derive its patients. The dummy catchment had to be socioeconomically, ethnically and culturally similar to the service area of the Hill–West Haven Division.

Our approach to creating a dummy catchment required three complementary, successive steps. The first was a gross descriptive overview of the metropolitan area that combined field observations with 1967 census data, historical sources and urban renewal literature.

The overview revealed that the Hill, while similar in most population and socioeconomic characteristics to other low income residential neighborhoods in New Haven, was unique in its racial and ethnic composition and in some housing characteristics. Similarly, West Haven was significantly different from the eleven other suburban towns, being the largest, having the highest population density, the greatest proportion of non-whites, the lowest socioeconomic status and a population slightly older than the other towns. Finally, and perhaps most important, the catchment as a whole was unique as an urban wedge. No other inner city neighborhood lay contiguous with working class suburbs. A band of middle and upper middle income residential neighborhoods is consistently interposed between inner city and suburbs elsewhere in the metropolitan New Haven area.

These considerations made it clear that it would not be possible to match the catchmenting precisely with a continuous geographic unit elsewhere in the metropolitan area. By eliminating the tracts of West Haven with concentrations of commerce and industry, non-whites and the oldest housing, however, it became possible to delineate a base population that closely matched the characteristics of another suburban town, East Haven. The unique characteristics of the Hill, however, precluded selecting a single inner city neighborhood as a comparative population sample. Smaller units of analysis than neighborhoods were required if the Hill population was to be adequately matched with another inner city sample.

Having reached these general conclusions, we then moved to the second step where the selected areas were subjected to a careful unit by unit matching on a block-group basis for the inner city and a census tract basis for the suburbs. Matching was done using three key variables: total population, proportion of non-white population and socioeconomic index. In addition, two discrete variables contained in the composite index of socioeconomic status were used to control for the expected variations on these dimensions: the Overcrowding Index and the Normal Family Life Index. With the exception of population density and age structure, these five variables represented all the dimensions on which the Hill and West Haven were found to differ significantly from other areas.

As shown in figure 4–2, the results of this matching process is a

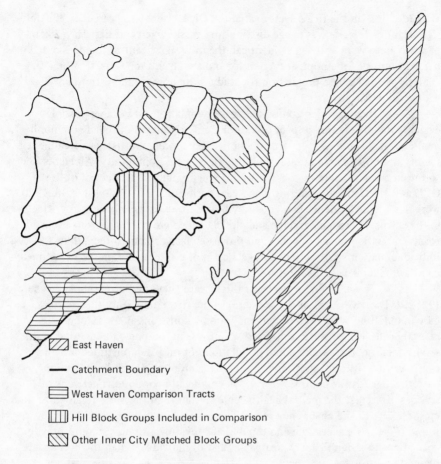

Figure 4-2. Hill-West Haven Division Catchment Area and Comparative Areas of Primary Service Region

mosaic on the map of the New Haven metropolitan statistical area. Neither the catchment nor the comparative populations represent a geopolitical unit in its entirety. This is unfortunate in that the political and social consciousness of a neighborhood or town may show a relationship to the utilization of mental health services. Since there were no comparable geopolitical units, however, this similarity was sacrificed for the best possible match of population characteristics.

Once the areas for study had been selected, we statistically tested the comparability of the populations in terms of both the selector variables and those included in the earlier ecological analysis. This was the third step in our creation of the dummy catchment. Except for the overcrowing index (eleven percent in the Hill versus seven percent in the non-Hill area) the inner city block groups were identical on the five selector variables. Of the remaining variables, the only significant difference was in age distribution. West Haven and East Haven comparative areas were also nearly identical, the only significant differences noted being in terms of the population density and age structure. Thus, the three stage analysis yielded a base population for study quite homogeneous from an ecological perspective.

By generating comparable base populations, it became possible to evaluate the differential impact of a catchmented, federally funded community mental health center as opposed to a non-catchmented, multiservice treatment facility upon the use of mental health services in the community. All admissions to the emergency room of the YNHH and the psychiatric services of both the GCD and HWH divisions during a one-year period, July 1, 1969—June 30, 1970, were recorded. Residence was coded by block group in the city or census tract in the towns. Sociodemographic and clinical data were obtained from admission forms and patient charts, coded, and processed using standard techniques. Individual patients rather than contacts, from the catchment and non-catchment areas were identified and compared.

The substantive results of this research have been presented elsewhere. [22, 23] They will be summarized here. In the first study, only the controlled base populations were used. Emergency room admissions at the catchmented mental health center were contrasted with those at the non-catchmented multiservice facility. The catchmented population not only demonstrated a significantly greater utilization of services, but also exhibited a shift in utilization patterns towards the comprehensive, systematic and continuous network of services offered at the mental health center rather than the more fragmented and episodic care of the emergency room. The catchmented mental health center was found to be more accessible and capable of providing a similar amount of care per patient to a significantly greater number of individuals than the non-catchmented multiservice treatment facility (tables 4–6 and 4–7.) These differences were most pronounced in comparisons between inner-city and suburban areas.

A second study combined both descriptive epidemiologic and ecologic approaches in order to measure whether catchmenting per se was associated with a diminution of bias in the allocation of mental health services both to disadvantaged groups and to certain clinically defined populations at risk. Initially, all admissions to the non-catchmented facility and the catchmented center were compared, irrespective of whether they came from the controlled population areas. Consistently greater representation of socially disadvantaged groups was found in the patient population of the catchmented center. When the same analyses were repeated using only the controlled base populations, however, these differences no longer emerged. Socially disadvantaged groups were found to be relatively overrepresented in the patient populations of both the actual catchment and the dummy catchment. These findings indicated that an urban wedge catchment placed an implicit control on service demand resulting in greater utilization of services by populations previously denied them.

Table 4-6. Catchmenting and the Use of Mental Health Services.

	Volume of Service Provided				
	Catch-mented Population	*Non-Catch-mented Population*			
Ratio of ER Contacts/ Patients Seen	1.37	1.40	$\bar{X}^2 = .4;$	d.f. = 1	N.S.
Ratio of Outpatient Treatment/ Evaluation Time	1.68	1.50	$\bar{X}^2 = 2.14;$	d.f. = 1	N.S.
Mean Number of Individual Therapy Hours	8.7	8.5	$Z = .036$		N.S.
Mean Inpatient Stay	50.0 days	47.4 days	$Z = .057$		N.S.

While the direct incentive for these studies was an interest in assessing the impact of catchmenting on delivery of mental health services, the approach can be applied to study the impact of a different organization of services or treatment ideology upon service utilization. Assuming that center 1 delivers service for community A and center 2 for community B and that the amount of services delivered and consumed by both communities can be measured, then one can then go on to design a relatively simple study model so long as efforts have been made to insure that A equals B and 1 is not equal to 2 (i.e., the communities are the same but centers are different). When this holds true, differences in the amount of services consumed by two communities or the outcome of such services (if one is interested, for example, in comparing different treatment ideologies) might be explained by the impact of the centers rather than by community demands.

Social area analysis, which is based upon the use of census data, is

Table 4-7. Patterns in the Use of Mental Health Services

	Catch-mented Population		*Non-Catch-mented Population*			
	No.	*%*	*No.*	*%*		
ER Only	258	25	218	33		
ER + MHC	225	22	161	24	$\bar{X}^2 = 14.7;$ d.f. = 2; P < .001	
MHC Only	535	53	291	43		
	rate/1000		*rate/1000*		*Z-score*	*P*
ER Only	5.8		4.8		.015	N.S.
ER + MHC	5.1		3.5		.111	N.S.
MHC Only	12.0		6.4		4.21	< .001

helpful in addressing such issues.[12, 24] The technique assumes that most of
the behavior of residents living in a geographically defined area can be explained
(and thereafter controlled for research purposes) in terms of "social rank" (social
class, occupation, education, income, life style (e.g., family committed life in
single dwelling-unit areas, working couple life in apartment house areas) and
ethnicity. This technique formed the basis of the studies reported as well as work
by Wolford et al. assessing the impact of the service organization on the delivery
of care.[25]

THE NEED-DEMAND CONTINUUM IN
MENTAL HEALTH SURVEYS

In the preceding section, we made use of census data to explore aspects of the
relationship between the need and the demand for service. Let us now consider
the use of a community survey as a vehicle for identifying commonalities and
differences between the "severely psychologically impaired" and those who
"seek" or "demand" care. In this way we should be able to not only isolate
various population characteristics that act as corollaries of mental health center
use, but also measure the contribution that these social, economic and mental
health variables make in determining who becomes a patient.

To accomplish this, it is necessary to combine into a single data base
the results of a mental health survey and a one-year sample of all admissions.
From a theoretical point of view, if admission to the center is random, then both
populations should be similar and any differences between the two samples may
be attributed to the selection process. If the distribution of symptoms or impaired mental status in both populations can be controlled, one may attempt to
investigate other variables correlated with entry to the service system or with
rejection of entry at the same level of "needs." An example of such investigation
conducted in the Hill–West Haven catchment area follows.

The Method

The Setting: The mental health catchment area being studied has a
population of approximately 72,000 in metropolitan New Haven. It includes
a changing inner city section of 22,000 and a more stable industrial town of
50,000. The area represents a cross section of the New Haven population and
includes all ethnic, racial and socioeconomic groups. The catchment is served by
a federally funded community mental health program, the Hill–West Haven
Division of the Connecticut Mental Health Center. The clinical program of the
Division includes a full range of mental health services structured to assure continuity of services. Team mechanisms are used to coordinate patient care.

The Community Survey: Between July 1967 and January 1968,

Myers and his colleagues surveyed a representative sample of adults from the catchment. The sample consisted of residents 18-years or more old, selected at random from each of 936 households. Respondents were reinterviewed in 1969 and 1970. Upon both occasions, information was gathered: (1) basic demographic variables, (2) physical health status, (3) mental health status, (4) social and instrumental role performance, and (5) life crises occuring during the year preceding the interviews. The representativeness of the sample was checked by comparing 1967 survey data with data from a special census of the New Haven SMSA conducted in the spring of 1967. The survey population was found to be sociodemographically comparable to the census population.

Mental health status was measured by an instrument which MacMillan developed and Gurin et al. later modified. It utilizes a list of 20 psychiatric symptoms that have been developed into an index of mental status. Previous research indicates that relatively low scores identify individuals with major psychological problems. Individuals scoring 66 and lower were classified as "very impaired psychologically," those scoring between 67 and 76 as "moderately impaired," and those scoring 77 and above as "unimpaired." In the current study, the sample was dichotomized in order to differentiate the very impaired from all other survey respondents. Sixteen percent of the sample fell into this category.

Data Analysis: A one-year sample (1969–1970) of patient admissions from the catchment, truncated so that the age range of both survey and patient samples corresponded, was selected for analysis. This yielded a patient sample of 808. A group of 182 patients aged 14–19 was excluded.

The study design called for comparing the characteristics of the patient population with those of the survey population. Survey data from 1969 were used for individuals interviewed in both 1967 and 1969. Where respondents refused to be reinterviewed, had moved without forwarding address, died or become senile, 1967 survey data were used. Preference was given to 1969 data because they coincided with the data on patient admissions. Six survey respondents who became center patients in 1969 or 1970 were excluded from the survey data base in order to eliminate overlap.

In the first comparison of the survey and patient samples it became clear that the age composition of the samples differed significantly. The survey sample had a mean age of 46 compared to 32 for the patients. For the subsequent analysis, therefore, the samples were divided into three age subgroups (20–29, 30–49, 50+).

A chi square test was then run separately for each of the subgroups on the basic sociodemographic characteristics of the CMHC and survey samples. Comparisons made were as follows:

1. Between the CMHC sample and the full survey sample to identify variables with differing distributions among patients and non-patients from the same geographic area.

2. Within the survey sample, between those classed on the Gurin score as very impaired and the rest of the population, to identify variables associated with psychiatric symptomatology in the community.
3. Between the CMHC sample and the very impaired subsample to identify those variables with differing distributions among center patients and psychologically impaired persons in the community.

Since the various characteristics studied are not entirely independent, the relationship between population characteristics, mental health center use and psychological impairment was further studied through the application of multivariate technics. In the multivariate analyses, both patient and survey populations were combined. Data were comparable with the exception of the assessment of psychological impairment. Drawing upon the literature related to clinical corollaries of the Gurin-MacMillan score, we devised a system for categorizing the patient population that was comparable with the "high symptom level—lower symptom level" dichotomized classification used for survey respondents.

CMHC patients were categorized as lower symptom level if (1) they were diagnosed as drug dependent (APA #304-304.99) (2) they were treated at the Drug Dependent Unit of CMHC and not assigned a diagnosis, or (3) none of the conditions defining high symptom level held true. CMHC patients were classified as having a high symptom level if they (1) had an APA diagnosis in one of the following ranges: 290-298, 300-301, 305-306, 309-310, (2) were treated on an inpatient unit at CMHC during 1969 and 1970, (3) were referred to CMHC from another inpatient facility or unit, or (4) were referred from CMHC to an inpatient unit.

To determine the interrelationship among the various sociodemographic variables, mental health status, mental health center use and distance from the center, and to test the validity of previous observations, a factor analysis was performed. The analysis was based on the samples of 938 survey respondents and 808 patients. In a second analysis to determine which items best predict mental health center use, a stepwise multiple regression technique was applied with mental health center use as the dependent variable.

Results of the Univariate Analysis

Age: As previously noted, the age distribution of the survey and patient populations differed significantly. A series of 2 × 3 chi square analyses were used to explore the relationships among age, MHC use and psychological impairment. The results, presented in table 4-8, indicate a proportionally greater representation of 20–29 year olds among the patient population as compared with either the community at large (full survey) or the very impaired subsample. There is no indication of an association between age and psychological impairment. Taken together, these findings suggest that age operates as a predictor of

Table 4-8. Age, Mental Health Center Use and Psychological Impairment

Ages	CMHC Users		Full Survey Sample		Impaired Sub-Sample		Unimpaired Sub-Sample	
	No.	%	No.	%	No.	%	No.	%
20–29	447	56	195	22	37	25	158	20
30–49	272	34	330	36	47	31	283	36
50+	83	10	403	42	66	44	337	44
Totals	802		928		150		778	

Results of 2 X 3 Chi Square Tests:

CMHC vs. Survey	$X^2 = 307.6$;	df = 2; p < .001
Impaired vs. Unimpaired	$X^2 = 2.05$;	df = 2; NS
CMHC vs. Impaired	$X^2 = 115.7$;	df = 2; p < .001

MHC use independent of mental health status. To minimize bias, therefore, age specific analyses were subsequently performed.

As the survey table indicates (table 4-9), the age specific analyses show certain populations to be high risk groups both in terms of psychological impairment and greater use of mental health center services. Included were non-whites and separate/divorced persons from all age groups, welfare recipients (age 20–49), individuals from the lowest economic strata (30–49), and persons with less than a high school education (30–49). While they are overrepresented as patients when compared with the population at large, higher utilization is con-

Table 4-9. Relationship between Population Characteristics, Mental Health Center Use and the Distribution of Psychiatric Symptomatology in the Community

Overrepresentation in the patient population consistent with the distribution of psychiatric symptomatology in the community:
  a. Non-whites
  b. Separated/divorced individuals
  c. Welfare recipients (20–49)
  d. Class 5 individuals (30–49)
  e. Individuals with less than a high school education (30–49)

Overrepresentation in the patient population independent of the distribution of psychiatric symptomatology in the community:
  a. The unemployed
  b. Individuals living alone (20–49)
  c. Individuals with no major religious affiliation (20–49)
  d. Class 5 individuals (20–29)
  e. Males (20–29)
  f. Females (50+)
  g. Individuals with less than a high school education (20–29)
  h. Individuals not currently married

sistent with a higher prevalence of psychological impairment in these groups. The seeming overrepresentation might more accurately be described as a concordance between the need for care and the receipt of service. Conversely a discordant relationship exists for certain groups such as middle aged women, persons under 30 with low incomes, and older individuals with less formal education. These groups utilized the center in significantly smaller numbers than would be expected if there was a linear and absolute relationship between the level of psychiatric improvement in the community and admission to treatment.

It is also possible to identify populations characterized by overrepresentation in terms of center admissions in the absence of appreciable evidence that the defining characteristic has a special relationship to mental health status. Stated another way, there are identifiable groups of individuals more likely to seek and receive psychiatric care from a mental health center than might be anticipated solely on the basis of the epidemiologic distribution of illness in the community. Young males, older females and young people from social class 5 exhibit this pattern. So also do individuals, regardless of age, who are currently unmarried, unemployed, living alone and without major religious affiliation. This latter constellation indicates the existence of a state of anomie or social disconnectedness not tapped by symptom inventories that acts as a strong initiator of help-seeking behavior.

Results of the Multivariate Analysis

The item-by-item univariate analyses revealed that the penetrance of the population characteristics included was incomplete and consequently age specific or non-linear. It was decided, therefore, to apply multivariate techniques both to confirm and explicate the initial observations.

A factor analysis was undertaken to determine the interrelationships among the variables included in the previous item-by-item analyses. From among the twenty-five individual variables analyzed, seven factors were extracted accounting for 57 percent of the variance. CMHC patienthood, loaded above .28 on only one of the seven factors. This factor, presented in table 4-10, also loads higher than any other on psychological impairment. Thus, patienthood describes the young person of low socioeconomic status who is unattached, isolated, resides in close proximity to the center and exhibits significant psychological impairment.

A stepwise multiple regression analysis was then employed to determine the relative influence of the independent variables upon patienthood. All items which correlated above .15 with patienthood were included in the equation.

As table 4-11 indicates, six variables account for 38 percent of the variance. The results underscore the importance of age as the most powerful predictor of patienthood. The second, fourth and sixth items (unmarried status and no religious affiliation) as indexes of potential isolation account for the next largest variance, twelve percent; impaired mental status comes next, five percent; followed by unemployment, which accounts for the least amount of variance.

**Table 4-10. Principal Component Factor Loading:
CMHC Patienthood**

CMHC Patienthood	+.63
Non-white	−.60
Unemployed	+.57
Separated or divorced	+.54
Distance to CMHC	−.54
Welfare	+.52
Age	−.41
Single	+.40
Social class	+.40
Living alone	+.39
Impairment	+.32

Summary. Controlling for the prevalence of psychological impairment in the community enabled us to reexamine the question of equity of service from a new perspective. What initially appears as a simple bias favoring the allocation of care to disadvantaged groups and thus correcting imbalances in delivery of services, now emerges as a complex phenomenom. In certain instances the bias tends to bring into closer approximation the need for care and receipt of service, as reflected by the prevalence of psychological impairment in the community. In other instances the bias operates even in the absence of a demonstrable association between the psychological impairment and the population characteristic studied.

Indeed, as the multivariate analyses indicated, age emerges as the strongest predictor of patienthood, regardless of symptomatology or any sociodemographic characteristics. This center, presumably like many others, is used extensively by young people, whether or not they have psychiatric symptomatology. Equally important is the finding that the larger portions of patients than even impaired persons in the community are disadvantaged and isolated in many ways—not only unemployed, non-white and on welfare, but separated/divorced, single, living alone and unaffiliated with any major religious group. While the mental health center program may draw its patients from those with high symptomatology in the community, this factor is only one among many in determining who receives and who becomes a patient.

In the study, a community survey was used as the point of departure

**Table 4-11. Results of Regression of CMHC Patienthood and
Independent Variables**

Variable	Contribution to R^2	Cumulative R^2
Age in years (negatively)	.195	.195
Separated or divorced	.080	.275
Impairment of mental status	.051	.326
Single	.026	.352
Employed (negatively)	.019	.371
No major religious group affiliation	.007	.379

Multiple Correlation $(R) = .609$

in focusing on an operationally defined population at risk—persons from the catchment with high symptomatology. Studies of the Gurin Mental Status Index indicate that it discriminates significantly between groups of psychiatric patients and non-patients living in the community, individuals judged by clinicians to be psychiatrically impaired and those deemed unimpaired, and between hospitalized and non-hospitalized psychiatric patients. Thus, it represents a validated instrument for identifying individuals within the community exhibiting significant psychiatric impairment and provides a mechanism for identifying commonalities and differences between the psychologically impaired and persons from health services. With these data, the interaction among various population characteristics, patienthood and psychological impairment were explored to determine whether the bias observed in earlier studies favoring the allocation of mental health services to populations previously denied them is consistent with or independent of the epidemiologic distribution of illness in the community.

The study documents the complexity of the interaction between the clinical program of a mental health center and the community it serves. Previous observations, derived from studying elements of the need-demand continuum on the basis of census data were confirmed. In addition, high facility utilization was often found to be associated with the prevalence of symptoms in the community, particularly where the defining characteristics described socially disadvantaged status. A second set of variables correlated with mental health center use but not the prevalence of symptoms. By and large, these characteristics describe a societal disconnectedness not necessarily related to social status. Finally, certain groups within the community, particularly the elderly and middle-aged woman, were unrepresented as patients even though they were members of populations where the prevalence of mental disorder was reasonably high.

CONCLUSIONS

In the preceding pages, we have attempted to outline a strategy that permits a systematic study of the need-demand continuum. While the examples do not provide definitive answers concerning the true incidence and prevalence of mental disorder in the community or the concatenation of factors which eventuate in the transformation of a perceived need for care into an expressed demand for service, certain generalizations seem in order:

1. the community has a reservoir of potential cases far in excess of the number of patients currently being accommodated by the mental health service system studied;
2. various ecologic factors can be pinpointed that influence patterns of expressed demand in the community and account for differential use of the formal mental health service network;
3. those factors also tend to influence interaction with other elements of the

human resource matrix, which suggests the utility of viewing and studying the mental health system as a part of a larger system of human service delivery;
4. the importance of system connectedness becomes all the more important in that the actual demand for mental health care may be more strongly influenced by factors associated with disadvantaged social status and social isolation than by psychological impairment;
5. the responsiveness of the mental health service system, however, can be enhanced by clearly assigning service responsibility for a defined population of potential users and structuring programs to insure accessibility comprehensiveness and continuity.

The value of the ecologic and epidemiologic methods resides in their ability to address two basic evaluative questions that cannot be answered simply by counting admissions to existing mental health facilities: What is the extent of the unmet needs for mental health services in the community? What are the factors that direct potential clients to a mental health service system? Their limitations arise from the general confusion in psychiatry about what represents a case. While constraints are placed upon any methodologic approach where definitional problems exist, so long as this dilemma remains unresolved, more definitive answers to the questions posed above must wait.

Chapter Five

Development of Standards for Evaluation of Direct Patient Care

Gary L. Tischler

In the preceding chapter, attention was focused on assessing the interrelationship of need versus demand for mental health services from an ecologic and epidemiologic perspective. Such studies begin with the assumption that minimal benefit accrues to a particular community if large numbers of residents are either denied access to or seriously handicapped in obtaining care, even though a minority may have ready access to service of excellent quality.

The view of accessibility and equity as prime dimensions of quality receives less attention in patient care evaluation because it involves taking into account phenomena not entirely under the control of the provider and requires obtaining and analyzing data concerning the ecologic characteristics of a service area and the help-seeking behaviors of its inhabitants. Whether a person decides to seek help and the form of help sought depend not only upon the availability of treatment resources, their physical proximity and the psychological and monetary costs of seeking assistance, but also upon a host of psychosocial factors which influence the ways in which given symptoms are perceived, evaluated and acted upon.[1–3] Furthermore, concern for an entire population and service area requires evaluating the care received from several sources and given by many types of providers.[4–6] These dilemmas notwithstanding, access and equity can be sensitive indicators of provider performance.

Once the issues of access to care and the equitable distribution of services are addressed, however, there is still a need to determine whether actual levels of clinical practice in a community conform with current standards of "goodness" operative within a particular field or profession. The determinations involve identifying aspects of care that merit consideration and developing methods for distinguishing "good" care from "bad." This is no mean task. The process of care comprises a complex set of activities reflecting provider behaviors, client behaviors and client-provider interactions that, in turn, consist of many discrete elements influenced by a host of transcendent organizational and societal factors. Additionally, delineations of good versus bad care are most frequently temporary and conditional since they are derived from judgments reflecting orientations dominant at a given time and subject to change either as knowledge advances or as the scope of provider responsibility is redefined.

In attempting to meet these difficulties, the Psychiatric Utilization Review and Evaluation Project chose a patient-care assessment program operating in a general hospital as a model to build upon and modify for use in community mental health centers. The 761-bed Yale–New Haven Hospital has developed an assessment program to provide a sophisticated and economical analysis of clinical process. At its core is a patient classification scheme based on unique combinations of diagnostic and demographic characteristics. Empirical norms exist for each patient class. Initial screening by electronic data processing equipment identifies statistically-deviant cases for further review. A probability sample of non-deviant cases is also obtained for control purposes.

Once a case is chosen for review, detailed clinical information is abstracted from the patient's medical chart by paramedical personnel for evaluation according to preestablished diagnosis-specific criteria. These criteria were constructed by the medical staff. They specify the conditions under which a patient should be admitted to the hospital, procedures required by, consistent with or contraindicated by the diagnosis and requirements for discharge. The results of the evaluation are then used to determine the efficacy of the initial screening and the adequacy of the criteria used in the review. This feedback permits adjustments to be made in the criteria, so that cases with a high probability of needing review will continue to be identified by the screening program.

Several problems arise in attempting to transpose the Yale–New Haven system to a mental health setting. They stem primarily from controversy within the field mentioned previously, including the difficulty of achieving consensus as to what represents an illness condition, the influence that non-diagnostic parameters exert upon the allocation of elements of care, and the divergent expectations and definitions of success held by patient, family, therapist and (at times) society.

To compensate for these problems, a criterion-oriented approach was adopted that begins by reducing the care-giving process to a set of monotonic representations focusing initially upon qualitative rather than structural issues. The representations are phrased as value-equivalents that have the additional benefit of providing a referential context within which more precise delineations of good as opposed to bad patient care can be made. The value equivalents considered fundamental ingredients of quality care were appropriateness, adequacy and effectiveness. To be *appropriate* the allocation of specific components of care should be consistent with a set of parameters that establish admission standards. To be *adequate*, the care-giving process should include those methods which are consistent with and required by the presenting problem. The methods themselves should also be bounded by explicit standards defining legitimate clinical conduct. To be *effective*, care should be associated with the attainment of specified objectives in relation to the presenting problem.

CRITERIA AND THE QUALITY OF PATIENT CARE

Most broadly defined, criteria represent standards against which something can be measured. According to Donabedian's [7] usage, such standards may be either normative—derived from the opinion of professionals—or empirical—based upon the actual practices of such professionals. Both reflect the consensus of clinicians on the state of the art at a given time and represent the operational translation of clinical pragmatism into a set of rules for assessing the quality of patient care. Implicit standards and judgments are made explicit through establishing parameters to delimit what represents appropriate, adequate, and effective care.

Normative criteria are formulated on the basis of professional opinion around an ideal of what represents excellence in clinical practice. A number of methods have been used to develop such criteria. These include the judgment of highly qualified practitioners [8], textbooks and standard publications [9], expert panels [10–12] and polls of practitioners.[13, 14] Since such opinions, notions and pronouncements are likely to derive more from a body of legitimate knowledge and values than actual practice, their validity depends upon the extent of agreement concerning facts and values within a particular profession. As a result, questions have arisen about how relevant normative standards developed by one group can be to the practices of another. Similarly, dissatisfaction has been expressed about applying to general practice settings standards and criteria elaborated in academic centers.

Empirical criteria are formulated on the basis of actual patterns of care as shown by statistical analysis. They can be used to compare care in one setting with that in another or with statistical averages obtained from a number of similar settings. Since such criteria reflect demonstrable levels of care, they are likely to be more creditable and acceptable to practitioners-at-large and less subject to criticism as idealized constructs. There is, however, one major limitation to the use of empirical standards. Although the care-giving process may appear to be adequate in comparison with other situations, it can still fall short of what is attainable through the full application of current knowledge. Thus, it seems advisable to have empirical observation serve as standards only if a normative element of judgment is added. Ideally both normative and empirical sources should be drawn upon in evolving standards of care.

Criteria of Appropriateness

Criteria of appropriateness provide guidelines for admission to treatment services. These guidelines or requirements are generally developed by partitioning a patient population into clinically meaningful groups receiving similar patterns of care. Because of the extent to which diagnosis determines treatment for hospitalized patients, a first cut in general medicine is usually made on the basis of diagnosis. Partitioning is subsequently performed through identifying key descriptors (both within and across diagnoses) that lead to the formation of more homogeneous patient groupings. Descriptors in general medicine found to be useful include secondary diagnosis, surgical procedures, age and sex, with length of stay and intensity of care used as dependent variables.

In psychiatry, however, the relationship between diagnosis and treatment is far less absolute. Furthermore, the accuracy of clinical diagnoses, as measured by repeatability either over time or on the basis of observer consistency, has proven to be less than reliable.[15-20] If the partitioning of patient groups is to be done on the basis of diagnosis, a higher degree of reliability between a given clinical description and the diagnostic label applied must be attained.

Advances have been made to increase the reliability of diagnoses through the use of computer technology. Spitzer and Endicott describe a computer program for psychiatric diagnosis based on a logical decision-tree model similar to the differential diagnostic process used in clinical medicine.[21] Input data are age and sex plus information on current psychopathology and psychiatric history including psychopathology personality characteristics, academic occupational and interpersonal adjustment from age twelve up to the month prior to admission. Output consists of 44 official APA diagnoses from the 1952 nomenclature and two unofficial diagnoses: nonspecific illness with mild symptomatology and not ill. The program yields one diagnosis for each subject. In a validity study, computer generated diagnoses for 100 patients agreed with diagnoses supplied by clinicians as well as did a second set of diagnoses supplied by different clinicians on the same case.

Recently, there has been increased interest in achieving diagnostic consistency through the use of rating scales. The *Handbook of Psychiatric Rating Scales* offers a documented account of some of the principles of rating scale design and use, and contains descriptions, critiques and levels of reliability and validity of nineteen scales reported in the literature.[22]

Within the context of the PURE Project, a rating scale for the diagnosis of schizophrenia was developed and refined by Astrachan et al. from 461 case records with a diagnosis of schizophrenia and 211 case records with other diagnoses.[23] Of those diagnosed as schizophrenic 87.6 percent scored for schizophrenia on the scale. False positives among the group of non-schizophrenics were 15.6 percent. Additional support for the scale was obtained through: (1) statistical comparison of individual symptoms used in the scale with the diagnosis of schizophrenia, (2) a cross validational study with an active patient sample, (3) factor analysis and (4) multiple regression analysis. The overall results were encouraging in terms of the ability of the scale to distinguish schizophrenics from a variety of other types of diagnostic groups and to index schizophrenic patients in six different types of treatment settings.

An alternative to scaling is symptom categorization. Robins and Guze have described a five-phase process for establishing diagnostic validity in psychiatric illness.[24] The phases include clinical description, laboratory studies, delimitation from other disorders, follow-up study and family study. Feighner et al. applied the technique while developing diagnostic criteria for fourteen psychiatric illnesses.[25] To validate the diagnosis of alcoholism, four symptom categories were used: medical-psychiatric effects of drinking, drinking behaviors, socioeconomic effects of drinking and the attitudes of self and other towards drinking. A "definite" diagnosis is made when symptoms occur in at least three of the four categories, a "probable" diagnosis when they occur in only two.

While advances increasing the reliability of diagnoses have been made through the use of computer technology, the development of diagnostic rating scales and symptom categorization techniques, the experience of the PURE project suggests that, at this time, the most economical approach to formulating criteria of appropriateness in general psychiatry is through linking various measures of psychosocial, environmental and biologic functioning, including diagnosis, to broad treatment categories such as inpatient, partial hospitalization or outpatient care.

A single measure or area of concern may be selected as the focal point around which to construct the criteria. One center, for example, took suicidal behavior as a point of departure. They next raised the question: Where suicidal behavior is the presenting problem, under what circumstances should hospitalization occur? A set of criteria, any one of which should lead a clinician to consider the possibility of compulsory hospitalization was then expounded. (See figure 5-1).

It is equally possible to construct criteria of appropriateness around decision points that define more generally the circumstance under which a particular dispositional option should be exercised. Thus, the staff of a second center adopted a checklist consisting of items subsuming a number of psychological, biologic, situation and behavioral factors that were felt to merit consideration in decision making related to hospitalizing applicants for mental health services.

Figure 5-1. Criteria for the Hospitalization of Patients Exhibiting Suicidal Behavior

---

If the patient exhibited any of the following:
  a. current, clear suicide attempt
  b. a clear, lethal suicide plan
  c. a recent history of medically serious attempts
  d. suicidal thoughts, gestures, or attempts in association with delirium or psychosis
  e. recent marked progression in seriousness of thought or from thought to gestures
  f. expression of strong suicidal thoughts with intent without seeing another way out
  g. an expectation of hospitalization that cannot be changed at interview
  h. expectation of change in significant others due to suicidal behavior are not met nor can be changed appropriately
  i. precipitating factor cannot be changed or
  j. high risk social circumstances, was he hospitalized (compulsorily if necessary)?

Each item was rated on a four-point scale of intensity and assigned a weight in terms of importance. When rated of sufficient intensity, some items were weighted so they stood as the sole criteria for admission. Others had to appear in an item cluster, with the cluster serving as the criterion. Hospitalization was considered the appropriate disposition when a scale score of 12 or above was obtained. See figure 5-2.

   The statement of appropriateness in the previous criteria took the form of circumstances under which particular actions should be taken. At times, however, it may be advisable also to indicate the circumstances where a particular disposition might be inappropriate. For example, the appropriateness of admission to a long term, psychotherapeutically oriented group treatment program was stated in terms of criteria for inclusion or exclusion. See figure 5-3.

   As these illustrations indicate, criteria for the appropriateness of psychiatric treatment usually take into account a wide range of factors other than diagnosis. They may be formulated in terms of indications or contraindications. A single criterion may be presented as a requirement for admission or the criteria themselves may be used to establish parameters against which clinical judgment can be tested.

Criteria of Adequacy

   Criteria of adequacy focus upon the treatment process per se. They are intended to insure that at least minimal standards govern the implementation of a treatment program.

   The question of adequacy may be addressed from a programmatic perspective. For instance, the criteria defining the adequacy of treatment received in a detoxification program for problem drinkers with intact families not only established standards of conduct governing nursing and medical practice, but also addressed issues related to participation in AA and Al-Anon meetings, family nite and family therapy. A population-specific focus may also be adopted. In addressing the treatment of adolescents, the staff of the center began with the assumption that a therapeutic intervention could be judged adequate only when the parents were actively involved. They then went on to stipulate the conditions under which exceptions could be made. See figure 5-4.

   At times, however, it becomes useful to take a more microscopic look at the treatment process. At one center, a neurological examination or an examination by a neurological consultant was required for all hospitalized patients when the admission work-up revealed a history of fainting, periodic headaches, vertigo, seizures, head trauma, fugue states, episodic violence or impairment of consciousness, orientation or cognitive function. The staff of another center developed diagnosis-specific guidelines for the use of psychotropic medications. For each medication, maximal dose levels were established, time spans within which a medication regimen had to be reviewed were developed and a program for baseline and dequential laboratory studies formulated. The use of

Figure 5-2.   A Checklist Approach in the Development of Criteria for Hospitalization

Instruction to reviewers: 1) Rate each patient on each criterion as: none = 0, slight = 1, moderate = 2, extensive = 3, multiply the rating by the weight shown and enter the score on each criterion. Then sum scores on each criterion for total score. 2) Ratings are to be based on the patient's condition in the seven days preceding evaluation for hospitalization. 3) In applying the criteria, an item of reported behavior should be employed to arrive at a rating on the first criterion on the list to which it applies. *Do not use* the *same* item of behavior to score a criterion that falls later in the list. (E.g. suicidal behavior should not be used in rating criteria numbers 4 & 5).

	Weight	Score
1. Is there evidence of active suicidal preoccupation, in fantasy or thoughts of patient? _____	2	___
2. Have there been suicidal attempts or active preparations to harm self (i.e., buying a gun, etc.)? _____	4	___
3. Has the patient threatened to hurt someone else physically? (Limit to verbal threats only.) _____	2	___
4. Have aggressive outbursts occurred toward people? _____	4	___
5. Have aggressive outbursts occurred toward animals or objects? __	2	___
6. Has antisocial behavior occurred? _____	1	___
7. Are there evidences of impairment of such functions as reality assessment, judgment, logical thinking, and planning? _____	1	___
8. Does the patient's condition seem to be deteriorating rapidly or failing to improve despite supportive measures? _____	1	___
9. Are there physical or neurological conditions or a psychotic, disorganized state which require(s) hospitalization to initiate the treatment process? _____	2	___
10. Does a pathological or noxious situation exist among patient's family or associates that makes initiation of treatment without hospitalization impossible? *OR* does the patient's disordered state create such difficulties for family or associates that he has to be removed and hospitalized for their sake? _____	1	___
11. Are emotional contacts of the patient so severely limited or the habitual patterns of behavior so pathologically ingrained that the "push" of a structured hospital program may be helpful? (This criterion should not be applied to acute patients, but only to those who are so limited as to be unable to establish and maintain emotional contacts.)_____	1	___
12. Does evaluation of the patient's condition require the 24-hour observation and special evaluation that a hospital provides? (Including stabilization or re-evaluation of medication.) _____	4	___

A modification of criteria from Whittington HG: *Psychiatry in the American Community.* (New York: International University Press, Inc. 1966).

Figure 5–3. Criteria for Admission to Long-Term, Psychotherapeutically Oriented Group Therapy

---

A. Criteria for Exclusion if the patient has any of the following characteristics:
    1. diagnosis of organic brain syndrome (PDR Numbers 290.0 through 294.8)
    2. diagnosis of paranoid (PDR Number 301.0)
    3. acutely suicidal (PAS Suicidal Thoughts, Gestures, or Acts rated Marked)
    4. acutely homicidal (PAS Assaultive Acts rated Moderate or Marked)
    5. described as acutely psychotic in the Intake or Admission Note
    6. hallucinating (PAS Hallucinations rated Moderate or Marked)
    7. inappropriate affect (PAS Inappropriate Affect, Appearance, Behavior rated Mild, Moderate, or Marked)
    8. low intellectual development (PAS Intellectual Development rated Dull or Retarded)
    9. poor impulse control
   10. external factors (going to leave the area soon, etc.)
    was he excluded from consideration for long-term group treatment?
B. Criteria for Inclusion if the patient had any of the following problems:
    1. primary problem was interpersonal
    2. a personality disorder other than paranoia (PDR Numbers 301.1 through 301.89)
    3. severe dependency problems (PAS Dependency, Clinging rated Moderate or Marked)
    4. sociopathic (PAS Antisocial Acts, Attitudes rated Slight or higher)

    was he assigned to a long-term group, or if not, was an explanation provided?

ECT was limited to patients who failed to respond to other treatment intervention but still exhibited life threatening behavior.

These examples indicate that criteria of adequacy establish parameters of legitimate clinical conduct within the context of specific treatment modalities and provide guidelines that indicate both the treatment interventions required by a patient consistent with various diagnosed problems and the alternative intervention to be undertaken if the initial intervention proves unsuccessful. The criteria themselves may be population, problem, modality or program specific. They are intended to insure that the treatment process proceeds in a rational and systematic manner.

Criteria of Effectiveness

Criteria of effectiveness are intended to measure the success or lack of success of a particular treatment episode. The criteria themselves are stated in terms of intermediate goals that can realistically be achieved during the course of a treatment intervention. They may be formulated from a program-specific perspective. Thus, the effectiveness of a medication maintenance program for chronically ill psychiatric patients was measured in terms of the degree to which program involvement was associated either with the prevention or with the reduction of psychiatric hospitalization and/or acute exacerbations of psychotic states. The criteria of effectiveness for the alcoholism detoxification and rehabilitation program mentioned earlier included: (1) the resolution of concrete dilemmas-in-living such as legal, financial, housing or employment problems, (2) improved family relations, (3) a more stable work record, where applicable and (4) the ability to control drinking over progressively longer time spans.

Figure 5-4. Exceptions for Parental Involvement in the Treatment of Adolescents

All records should include a statement about whether parents were involved, and, if not involved, an explanation why. Parents need not be involved if—
- The adolescents life situation is not chaotic
- The minor is emancipated, i.e.,
    a. out of the home for six months
    b. self sufficient
    c. not legally truant
        (The history of emancipation should be recorded including duration of current living arrangement and frequency and nature of contact with family.)
- The clinician feels that parental involvement during initial intake would preclude development of a therapeutic alliance, he may defer contact with both parents or one of them.

Alternatively, it is possible to approach the question of effectiveness from a patient-specific perspective. The criterion itself can be broadly stated to incorporate highly individualized goals as measures of effectiveness:

> At the time of admission, the intrapersonal, interpersonal and social problems with which the patient presented were clearly articulated. A problem-specific treatment plan was then formulated. At the time of discharge, significant improvement was recorded in the problem areas noted.

When a criterion is so broadly stated, the individualized measures must be quite specific. Thus, there is a need to define presenting problems in operational terms, develop terminal goals towards which therapeutic change can be directed and establish an ongoing system for measuring the direction and magnitude of change. An individualized goal achievement approach is routinely used by behavioral therapists.[26] It has also been used in assessing the effectiveness of drug therapies under the rubric of the eradication of "target symptoms."[27] Kirusek and Sherman have developed an extremely sophisticated method for setting up (prior to treatment) a measurable scale for each patient-therapist goal and specifying, for each patient, a transformation of overall goal attainment into a standardized T-score.[28]

One center applied the goal achievement model in a somewhat global fashion to assess the effectiveness of a neighborhood service center program. They began by constructing a problem inventory based upon a classificatory schema developed at Lincoln Hospital.[29] Major problem categories and problem subtypes were then defined: The discrete services offered at the center were also labeled and defined. Illustrations of this approach are provided in figures 5-5, 5-6 and 5-7.

When these interventions were undertaken, an action plan was to be formulated consistent with the problems catalogued in the inventory. The effectiveness of the intervention was measured in terms of achieving goals related

Figure 5–5. An Example of the Problem Inventory

I. Formulation of the Problem.
   A. Statement of the problem.
      1. Is there an overall statement of the patient's problem?

                    YES   NO

      2. Classify the problem(s) according to the following categories as defined in the accompanying manual:

FAMILY	PERSONAL	FINANCIAL
Marital	Recreation	Support
Recreation	Care	Extra Money
Care	School	Welfare Department
School	Medical	Social Security
Medical	Psychological	Workman's Comp.
Psychological	Social	Unemployment Ins.
Parent/Child	Parent/Child	Veteran's Admin.
		Union Benefits

COMMUNITY	LEGAL	HOUSING
Complaints	Rights	New
Action	Contracts	Tenants' Rights
	Civil	Utility Problem
	Criminal	Repairs

EMPLOYMENT	NOT CLASSIFIABLE
Need	Other: Explain briefly
Training	
Other	

Figure 5–6. Definitions from the Problem Inventory

FAMILY: This problem type covers any problem or request which directly affects another member of the client's family and the service rendered should be largely for that member of the family. If the problem could logically fall into another type (financial, legal, etc.) it should be classified as that type and not as a family problem. The following problem subtypes apply:

1. Marital problems involving a husband or a wife in their relationship to one another.
2. Recreation is needed for some member of the family. For example, after school activities, scouting, athletics.
3. Care or assistance is needed for some member of the family. This includes convalescent care for elderly persons, babysitting for small children, homemaker services, and limited specific requests for food and clothing. This category should not be used to cover care or help that is predominantly medical or psychiatric or that is suspected of being so.
4. School problems involving school-age children in the family. These may be academic or behavioral.
5. Medical problems or suspected medical problems, including medical care, health insurance, medicare, birth control, etc.
6. Behavioral or mental health problems involving any member of the family other than the client himself. This includes any problem suspected of being psychiatric and where normally a psychiatric referral would be considered. This category includes alcoholism and drug addiction.

Figure 5-7. The Classification of Direct and Indirect Services

I. DIRECT SERVICES

Intake: An interview concerning the appropriateness of availability of services including screening and referral services (for non-registered clients only).

Psychosocial Evaluation: A psychodiagnostic process which may include a medical history, a mental status examination, and an evaluation to ascertain the social situation of the individual, including such things as personal background, family background, family interactions, living arrangements, economic problems, and the formulation of future goals and plans.

Crisis Intervention: Services given to persons who are in an emergency situation and who present an immediate need for services.

Individual Treatment: Treatment by individual interview where the primary focus is the individual client. Includes counseling, supportive psychotherapy, relationship therapy and insight therapy.

Group Treatment: Treatment through the use of group dynamics or group interaction including group psychotherapy, group play therapy and psychodrama.

Expediting: The active intervention on a client's behalf in an attempt to secure or facilitate service to the client from any organization, agency, or individual outside of the mental health center. For a service to be coded as expediting, the worker must directly intercede as the client's advocate.

Concrete Service: Providing the client with direct help with such tasks as giving information in response to a request, filling out forms, transportation, delivery of medication, etc. This service differs from expedition in that in offering a concrete service, the worker tries to meet the client's needs directly rather than helping the client obtain the service elsewhere from another agency.

Home Visit Service: A service conducted in the temporary or permanent residence of the recipient to provide an objective assessment and help in meeting mental health problems, to assist families in utilizing community resources, and to provide direct service for patients or families.

II. INDIRECT SERVICES

Case Consultation: Assistance provided to staff of another agency or organization to help them provide better direct services to specific clients for whom they are responsible and in which mental health center staff do not assume responsibility for the client.

Program Consultation: Work with another community organization to assist them in planning and developing programs which they sponsor.

Administrative Consultation: Service provided to administrators in target groups or organizations with the goal of changing administrative structure or processes.

Community Organizing: Consultees are community residents, groups or organizations other than governmental and "official" service organizations. The goal is the facilitation of efforts of citizens/consumers to organize themselves to solve common problems, to gain increased power and control over institutions which affect their lives, etc. (e.g., Welfare Moms, Parents for an Elected School Board).

Public Information and Education: Activities focused on increasing knowledge and changing attitudes in the community at large and in specific target groups. It includes planned educational campaigns and routine responses to requests for information such as talks, news releases and pamphlets.

to the specific problems; furthermore, where an intervention was either unsuccessful or did not achieve preferred goals, the overall quality of the service was reevaluated on the basis of whether the goals were reformulated. The action plan was then modified or a new intervention undertaken.

Where so global a method for measuring effectivess is deemed inadvisable, scaled scores may be used as criteria that stipulated the conditions for discharge. Hogarty and Ulrich have developed such a scale which provides an objective measure of discharge readiness for hospitalized patients.[30] The Discharge Readiness Inventory consists of: (1) measures of observable ward behavior, (2) global prognostic judgments concerning potential for adjustment in the community and, (3) recommendations for the probable placement, amount of work and supervision required for patients judged ready for discharge. When factor analyzed, the inventory yielded four subscales, one of which proved a valid predictor of discharge readiness.

As these examples indicate, it is possible to formulate criteria of effectiveness from either a patient-specific or a program-specific perspective. In either case, however, attention must be paid to specifying endpoints that can be measured and to insuring that the measures exhibit a reasonable degree of concurrent and predictive validity.

A CRITERIA-ORIENTED APPROACH

Up to this point, our focus has primarily been upon what criteria are, what they are intended to measure, and the various forms they might take when formulated. Let us now turn to a more detailed consideration of the criteria-oriented approach adapted by the Psychiatric Utilization Review and Evaluation Project. The approach involves formulating standards, testing and validating the formulations and translating the criteria evolved from both normative and empirical sources into a format that facilitates individual case review

The Formulation of Criteria

The project's approach to criteria formulation began by calling together a group comprising both mental health practitioners representing all staff levels and clinical disciplines and social scientists. They were charged with developing standards against which the quality of patient care provided at a particular mental health center could be measured. The group started by examining various facets of the care-giving process through the careful review of patients' written records. The opinions and observations of the members in relation to the elements of care under review were discussed and recorded.

In addition to the written record, the committee also obtained data on the care-giving process by interviewing clinicians and through a search of relevant professional literature. In the first instance the committee met with individual practitioners to explore in detail clinical decision making. Emphasis was placed upon information requirements and the transformation of information into intervention strategies. From these interviews, a semistructured protocol was developed for further inquiry into various aspects of the therapeutic process through focusing upon the standards applied by individual clinicians in judging the adequacy of their own performance. In the second instance, an assistant was instructed to make a thorough topical literature review on the element of care under study. A bibliography was prepared together with abstracts and a summary report for presentation to the committee.

Empirical data were also solicited by the group to obtain a clearer picture of the clinical practices of the institution. This task involved the statistical analysis of aggregate data on the use of mental health services during a given time period. For example, it was found that first-break schizophrenics were likely to be placed on phenothiazines and remain in hospital for a three-month period. This represented the statistical norm for the institution and could therefore be considered as an empirical standard. Cases where the patient was discharged in one day or did not receive ataratics were examples of potentially aberrant (statistically deviant) care that should be explored in greater detail.

Special studies were also used to examine in more detail discrete aspects of the care-giving process. One example involved the epidemiologic study of the allocation of mental health services. The question addressed was whether demonstrable bias existed in the allocation of services to socially disadvantaged groups such as lower socioeconomic individuals, minority group members or welfare recipients. The results indicated a consistently higher utilization of the center reflected in overall admission rates than would be anticipated on the basis of the population characteristics of the area. On the other hand, the entry bias favoring disadvantaged groups was blunted when the internal movement of patients was examined. For example transfers of low socioeconomic individuals, minority group members and welfare recipients to the center's psychotherapy program were consistently lower than to either its drug abuse or inpatient/partial hospitalization services. These findings indicated the existence of a distributive bias, running counter to the entry bias, that had to be addressed as the group attempted to formulate standards related to the allocation of treatment services.

The information obtained from case review, interviews with clinicians, literature review, statistical analyses and special studies provided the group a data base derived from both normative and empirical sources. While these data were subject to interpretation by various members, the group served as a catalyst by forcing each participant to articulate clearly the pertinent factors influencing individual judgments. In this way, assumptions were called into question, and the influence of personal and professional biases upon definitions of "goodness" and "badness" were subjected to scrutiny. As a result, it was possible to translate implicit values and norms into explicit standards that could then be tested and validated.

The Testing and Validation of Criteria
While information derived from both normative and empirical sources was used to formulate the criteria, the standards themselves of necessity ultimately reflected normative judgments. This situation poses several problems in the mental health area. Generally, mental health practitioners are biased. They

have clear preferences for particular therapeutic modalities, prefer to deal with certain kinds of patients and problem areas and exclude others. When these considerations are superimposed upon the reality that there is currently no agreed upon definition of either mental health or illness, a need exists to test and validate the criteria being adopted. The second stage of the criterion-oriented approach used by the PURE Project, therefore, involved testing the normatively derived standards by pattern analysis, special study and follow-up study.

Special Pattern Analysis. It is often assumed that a specific psychiatric problem will lead to the need for specific components of care, including whether an individual is to become an inpatient or outpatient, the (service) unit of treatment, the frequency of utilization, whether family, group or individual therapy is to be administered, the specific type of drugs that are indicated, and the place to which the patient is ultimately referred.

Under certain circumstances it may be that psychiatric diagnosis, according to the American Psychiatric Association manual, will describe the patient's condition sufficiently well that it alone will be adequate to determine a specific mode of care. More frequently, however, other factors than the diagnosis alone will be necessary in order to describe the patient's psychiatric problem, including specific symptoms (e.g., suicide attempt) age, psychiatric history and the method by which the disturbed behavior is normally dealt with (e.g., by family, church, police, AA).

In addition, a wide variety of factors which depend not upon policies of the psychiatric institution but upon the patient's life style may influence the degree to which the patient is able or willing to use the institution: the character of interaction between patient and clinical staff and the degree to which influences outside the institution (such as family, police and work situation) influence the relationship between patient and clinical staff.

Moreover, in simply identifying the variety of patterns of care that occur in a mental health center, we need to discriminate on clinical grounds among typologies of care, according to variables which identify relevant characteristics of psychiatric history, specific symptoms and pertinent behavioral manifestations of symptoms such as may require special treatment (e.g., suicide attempt, drug or alcohol problem), for various socioeconomic and demographic characteristics of patients and their families.

The overall task is to describe the major typologies of care according to the specific characteristics of patients which predetermine that a group of patients will become relatively homogeneous in relation to the various components of their psychiatric care. For example, it is likely that individuals who have a similar major diagnosis, age, sex, history of psychiatric hospitalization and socioeconomic level may receive very similar treatment—treatment which, in turn, sharply distinguishes them from other homogeneous groups of individuals who tend to receive different types of treatment.

Thus, pattern analysis can serve the dual purpose of identifying homogeneous groupings of patients receiving similar patterns of care and determining whether these observed patterns conform to the normative standards established by the group. Using length of stay as the dependent variable, we found that the major factors affecting deviation from usual patterns of care included social class, town of residence, age and admitting diagnosis. For example, one homogeneous group comprised patients in Hollingshead and Redlich's social classes 1–4 between the ages of sixteen and twenty residing in the suburban New Haven area, with an admitting diagnosis of functional psychosis. Since a diagnosis of functional psychosis in an adolescent is a criterion for hospitalization, the analysis confirmed that, for this group of patients, observed practices conformed to normative standards.

Special, Outcome and Follow-Up Studies. A second method for empirically testing normative standards involves the use of special studies, outcome studies and follow-up studies. Such studies enable investigators to check expert opinion regarding quality of care against what actually happens to patients both while they are within and after they leave a treatment setting. Specific questions related to discrete aspects of the care-giving process can be investigated. Relationships among patient attributes, characteristics of treatment and outcome measures of mental status, social adjustment, role performance and post discharge treatment can be documented.

Since these techniques will be dealt with subsequently in detail, we shall not pursue the subject here. Suffice it that the techniques provide data which can not only be applied to constructing and/or modifying criteria, but also to evaluating the relationship among institutional standards, institutional practice and postdischarge performance.

Organizing Criteria for Use in Individual Case Review

The final stage of the criteria-oriented approach involves translating the criteria evolved from both normative and empirical sources into a format that facilitates individual case review. Let us take as an example the transformation of criteria related to appropriateness for day hospitalization into a case abstract format as an example.

The first step involved the delineation of the modes of admission. Two modes were identified, direct admission and transfer. Separate criteria were then developed for each:

Criteria	*Check List Items*
The initial question establishes the set being considered.	Was patient admitted directly to a day hospital unit?
The first set of criteria state: Day hospitalization is an appropriate alternative to full hospitalization	If YES,

Criteria	Check List Items

WHEN

the degree of psychopathology or the magnitude of a life crisis are of sufficient intensity to require a major intervention involving either the use of large doses of psychotropic medications or extensive environmental manipulation

Is there evidence presented that the patient was exposed to a current stressful (crisis) situation that requires close collaboration of CMHC with any of the following: family, friends, employer or school?

WHERE

no major physical contraindications demanding hospitalization exist;

Does the record indicate that the patients were either psychotic or depressed and required immediate treatment with a high dosage of medication?

IF YES for either:

did the medical evaluation show him to be in good physical health?

adequate environmental supports are available to moderate evening and weekend activity.

was the family able to provide adequate support and ability to care for the patient evenings and weekends?

The second set of criteria state:

Does the record indicate that the patient required an intensive psychiatric diagnostic work-up that could be more easily accomplished if the patient were partially hospitalized?

partial hospitalization is an appropriate alternative to full hospitalization or ambulatory care when a diagnostic evaluation can be accomplished more expeditiously and economically.

Does the record indicate that the patient required an intensive medical diagnostic work-up that could be more easily accomplished if the patient were partially hospitalized?

The third criteria states:

Partial hospitalization is appropriate for non-psychotic individuals where the symptom configuration suggests the need for a degree of structure prior to entering an ambulatory care program.

Does the record indicate that the patient's treatment program was oriented primarily towards outpatient therapy but that due to the patient's mental status (depression, psychomotor retardation, lack of plans) the patient needed a structured program in order to "get along?"

Once again, the set being considered must first be established.

Was the patient transferred from 24-hour hospitalization to day hospital status?

The criteria of appropriateness for transfer from 24-hour hospitalization to day hospitalization are:

IF YES,

Criteria	*Check List Items*
Measurable improvements during inpatient stay with an associated need for a transitional experience from full hospital to ambulatory care	Does the record indicate that the patient improved during his initial 24-hour hospitalization but still needed to spend a significant amount of time in the hospital program for any of the following reasons: mental status, nature of medication, need for a structured program, completion of discharge planning?
BECAUSE	
psychological functioning is still too tenuous	
medication regime has not yet been stabilized	
discharge planning is not complete	
adequate environmental supports are not yet in place.	

As the example suggests, the transformation takes the form of a series of questions requiring "yes-no" discriminations. The example itself represents but one of 110 items included in the abstract. Figure 5–8 illustrates the major areas covered. The format is constructed as a decision tree which measures the logic and consistency of the evaluative, treatment and disposition processes.

CONCLUSION

The basic elements of the criterion approach used by the Psychiatric Utilization Review and Evaluation Project consist of: (1) review of the care-giving process by a group of expert clinicians, (2) formulation of criteria and their transformation into a decision tree mechanism for assessing the quality of patient care, and (3) validation of the criteria through pattern analysis and follow-up studies.

Obviously, a set of standards cannot be imposed upon an institution where the "state of the art" is such that great variation exists both in the definition of what represents mental disorder or mental health and in the clinical approach to patient care. Rather, the function of a criterion-oriented approach is to ascertain whether the care given corresponds to the manifest goals of a service institution as formulated in a set of standards or guidelines related to the quality of patient care.

Where a criterion-oriented approach is used, implicit norms must be translated into explicit standards. These standards can then be used to detect not only cases where patient care deviates from desired norms but also cases where patient care has conformed to treatment standards yet the outcome has been unsatisfactory. As a result, the use of criteria and a criterion approach provides a vehicle for clarifying issues related to patient care that are now conceptually unclear and for monitoring the quality of care given by a wide variety of service institutions.

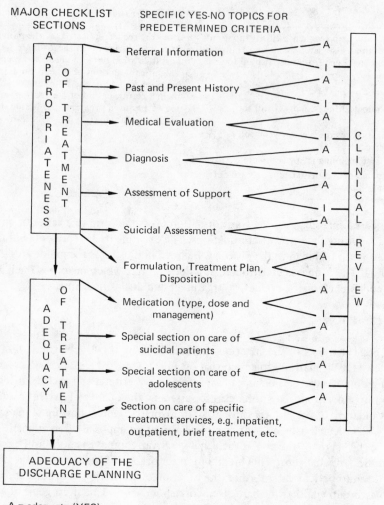

MAJOR CHECKLIST SECTIONS

SPECIFIC YES-NO TOPICS FOR PREDETERMINED CRITERIA

APPROPRIATENESS OF TREATMENT

- Referral Information — A / I
- Past and Present History — A / I
- Medical Evaluation — A / I
- Diagnosis — A / I
- Assessment of Support — A / I
- Suicidal Assessment — A / I

ADEQUACY OF TREATMENT

- Formulation, Treatment Plan, Disposition — A / I
- Medication (type, dose and management) — A / I
- Special section on care of suicidal patients — A / I
- Special section on care of adolescents — A / I
- Section on care of specific treatment services, e.g. inpatient, outpatient, brief treatment, etc. — A / I

CLINICAL REVIEW

ADEQUACY OF THE DISCHARGE PLANNING

A = adequate (YES)
I = inadequate (NO)

Figure 5-8. A Simplified Decision Tree for Individual Case Review

Chapter Six

The Application of Criteria in Assessing Direct Patient Care

Phillip B. Goldblatt

As an approach to patient care appraisal, individual case review is strongly rooted in medical tradition. The education of physicians initially relied heavily upon an apprentice model. Students would follow a practicing physician and learn the trade both by observation and by the gradual assumption of responsibility for clinical tasks under their mentor's supervision. In the traditional medical curriculum that operated in the United States from the time of the Flexner Report until the 1960s, elements of apprenticeship were incorporated into clinical clerkships during the third and fourth years of training. While it was presumed that the methods taught were appropriate and would be applied by other clinicians in similar situations, case conferences were included in the curriculum to balance potential idiosyncratic learning resulting from reliance, solely upon dyadic teaching methods. During such conferences, the student would present a particular case before a group of clinicians who would then discuss issues related to the appropriateness, adequacy and effectiveness of care being provided. The case conference, including its strong educative thrust, represent the prototype for individual case review.

Individual case review involves scrutiny, usually by a committee of peers, of the care provided a particular patient at a specific mental health center. There are two possible chronological approaches to individual case review, *retrospective* and *concurrent.*

Retrospective review is essentially an educative process. Since the patient has already been discharged, the review will probably prove of little direct benefit to him. It can, however, help to identify particular clinicians whose performance deviates significantly from institutional standards and also to identify issues related to the care-giving process that may substantially contribute to policy-making aspects of the utilization review process.

Concurrent review is conducted while the patient is still in treatment. Consequently, it is possible to monitor the actual care a patient is receiving. Such questions can be raised as whether the patient's condition has been properly diagnosed and treated, whether there is adequate communication between patient and provider and whether the treatment plan (including discharge planning) has adequately tapped all the resources required to maintain the person after discharge.

A particular form of concurrent review which merits specific attention is *extended duration review*. Continuous extended duration review is a major concern of insurors and is a condition of participation according to the Medicare formulation. This type of review requires that the records of all patients who have stayed in a facility for a period defined by the institution as extended duration, be reviewed to determine need for continued treatment. The definition of extended duration may be formulated by the institution. It can be a single limit for all patients or can be individually based on categories such as disease entities or particular treatment programs. Decisions and discussions during such reviews are usually focused to facilitate some final judgment as to whether a particular patient should or should not receive continued care. Thus, the primary thrust of extended duration review is the monitoring of facility over-utilization by clients whose stay exceeds their needs or who may appropriately be treated in some other setting.

A THREE-LEVEL PROCESS FOR INDIVIDUAL CASE REVIEW

As previously noted, the task of individual case review can be materially enhanced through the use of criteria-oriented approaches. Within the context of the PURE Project, the pressure for explicating criteria and translating them into an appropriate format for performing individual case review led to the development of a multilevel chart review check list.[1] Over a two-year period, several such checklists were compiled and tested for utility. The original focused on the admissions-intake process. It was designed to assess the completeness of the information contained in the chart as well as the logic and consistency of the evaluation, treatment plan and disposition.

To test the reliability of the instrument in the hands of non-clinicians, sixteen charts were reviewed independently by having each non-clinician complete a chart review checklist. There was agreement on more than 80 percent of all items, including a final global rating of whether the care provided in a particular chart was excellent, adequate or poor. This level of agreement was obtained without benefit of training sessions or an operations manual. Such a high level of agreement suggested the possibility that non-clinicians might be able to do most of the review work especially if the checklist was revised to make more explicit areas requiring judgment.

To test this premise, the checklist was revised and a three-level approach adopted which permits non-clinicians to assess items related to the adequacy of care as well as the adequacy of information. Such a technique permits the maximal use of paramedical personnel, requires a minimum of special training and involves clinicians only in examining instances of care that have already been shown to deviate from the criteria adopted by the institution. An overview of the various levels of review with appropriate feedback is provided in figure 6-1.

Level 1: Record Room Review

The first level of review involves examination of charts on all patients and is accomplished by personnel in the record room. Its goal is to determine the completeness of the information in the chart. Reviewers are instructed to indicate whether each form required by the institution is present and complete in the patient's chart. Charts found not to meet the minimum standards of completeness are returned to the attending clinician for completion. An example of checklist items related to record room review is provided in figure 6-2.

Level 2: Non-Professional Review

The second level of review is performed by non-clinical personnel under the supervision of a mental health professional. This review is performed on a certain number of completed charts selected as having a high probability of needing more intensive review. For example, cases are selected from such categories as suicide while in treatment, acute schizophrenic patients not receiving psychotropic medication, certain long stay categories, etc.

The goals of second level review are—

1. To establish the adequacy of the information recorded in the chart for clinical review, and
2. To establish whether or not the treatment described in the chart meets the criteria of good patient care set forth in the checklist.

The judgment of adequacy of care at this level is fully operationalized and embodied in the "yes-or-no" discriminations required by the checklist. These evaluations by non-clinical personnel do not primarily involve subjective judgments and are, therefore, reliable. This level of review is thus intended to establish adequacy of clinical care, but only by conformity to normative standards of care represented in the criteria. Judgment of adequacy of care where it does not conform to these model standards is the function of the third level reviewer.

Level 3: Clinical Review

The third level occurs when violations of criteria are found by the non-professional reviewer. At third level review the chart is examined by a mental health professional to ascertain whether the violation indeed indicates aberrant or poor care. The results of this review can be used by the utilization review committee to suggest changes in clinical practice of therapists, changes in

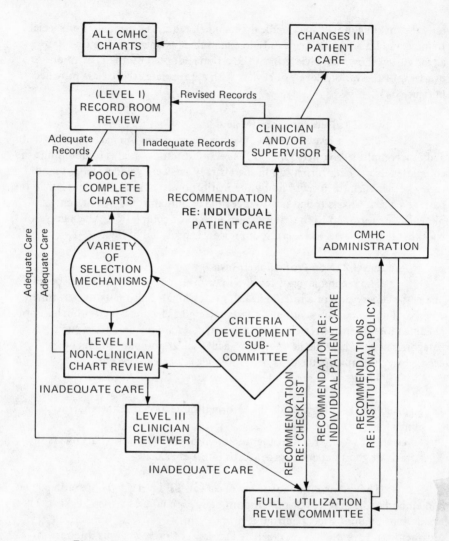

Figure 6–1.   Levels of Review

institutional or ward policies or revision of the criteria themselves. Thus, level 3 review also provides a continuing test of whether the checklist criteria are effective in discriminating between adequate and inadequate patient care.

The Interaction between Non-Professional and Clinical Review

Perhaps it would be useful to provide an example of the interaction between second and third level review. We shall focus on a patient admitted to outpatient brief treatment. The checklist raises the following questions:

Figure 6-2. Chart Review Checklist

Level 1—Records Room Review[1]

I. *Identification*

Patient's initials: _____

Sex: ___ Birthdate: _____ Race: _____

Reviewer's Name: _____

Date of Review: _____

Chart Number: _____

First CMHC Admission: Yes   No

Date of Admission Reviewed: _____

Unit of Intake: _____

Unit(s) on which treated: _____

_____

II. *Format of Chart*

  .A. (APPLICABLE TO ALL PATIENTS) The following forms are required in all CMHC patients' charts with the exceptions indicated. Are they present and *completed* in this chart as required?

*1. MSIS Admission Form	Yes No
2. CMHC Supplement Form	Yes No
3. Initial Contact-Referral Form or ER Sheet	Yes No
*4. PER-C or MSER	Yes No
5. Clinical Transfer Form (if patient transferred within acute service, within continuing care unit in GCD, or from continuing care to inpatient or between corresponding treatment modalities in H-WH Division).	Yes No NA
*6. Dictated Admission/Transfer/Discharge Summary	Yes No
IF YES, was it executed within 30 days of initial visit?	Yes No NA
*a. Is Admission Diagnosis recorded?	Yes No
*b. Is Discharge Diagnosis recorded? (If patient was treated less than 30 days, one diagnosis can be considered as both admission *and* discharge diagnosis.)	Yes No
c. (If patient was treated more than six weeks, or treated in other than admission unit), are there both Admission/Transfer *and* Discharge Summaries in the chart?	Yes No NA
7. CMHC Change of Status Form indicating unit to which first assigned (if patient admitted to treatment at CMHC)	Yes No NA
8. Financial Form (if patient admitted to treatment at CMHC)	Yes No NA
9. Progress Notes (if patient is inpatient or was seen more than 30 days in outpatient unit)	Yes No NA

	YES	NO
1. Was patient treated in an outpatient brief treatment unit?	X	
2. If yes,		
a. Was (is) the goal(s) of the present contract defined?		X
b. Were the external precipitating factors defined?	X	
c. During the last year, was the patient at least 6 months without continuous psychiatric treatment?		X
d. If medication was given, were the target symptoms defined?		X

If the level 2 reviewer (non-professional paramedical personnel) indicated the answer to any question raised in item 2 a–d was no, then the chart would be forwarded to the third level where a clinician reviewer determines whether the treatment or choice of treatment was adequate.

For instance, second level review reveals that a patient was admitted to the brief treatment unit. Prior to admission the goal of the contract was not defined. The external participants were identified. During the past year the patient had not been six continuous months without psychiatric treatment. Medication was prescribed, but the target symptoms were not defined in the chart. Since three items were checked no, the chart was forwarded for third level review. The clinician reviewer considered the treatment program inadequate on the grounds that it paid insufficient attention to the patient's antecedent help-seeking behaviors or the nature of the primary problem—drug abuse. His judgment was that residential treatment or admission to a specialty unit for inpatient detoxification should have been the point of departure in this patient's treatment program.

The Revised Checklist

The final revision of the checklist, presented in appendix B, includes more than three hundred yes-no items. Not all must be answered for each patient. The items are organized into specific topics such as adequacy of referral information, past and present history, medical evaluation, assessment of support and formulation of treatment plan. There are also special sections relating to the care of suicidal patients and adolescents.

At present it would require the greatest number of items to examine the care of an adolescent with a history of previous psychiatric or medical care who had been treated in the past on several mental health center services and is currently suicidal or schizophrenic. It would take a skilled second level reviewer about an hour to read the chart and fill out the checklist and a third reviewer about 25 minutes to read the chart and comment upon the items selected for clinical review as well as upon overall adequacy. If the third level reviewer limits himself to commenting on the items checked as inadequate, his review time is much shorter.

The three-level approach employs procedures which move toward increasing the ease and the reliability of a review process. The use of predetermined selection mechanisms and preestablished criteria of adequate care permits the selection of cases with a higher probability of needing review than a randomly selected group of cases. Further, variations due to lack of structure and to idiosyncratic responses by reviewers are minimized. A recent study by Richardson [2] suggests that just the introduction of a list of items expected in the chart of the patient receiving the best clinical care might significantly increase the accuracy of medical audit.

Checklists such as the one described above also permit the use of non-clinicians to perform the bulk of the review. Mental health professionals whose time is expensive are utilized to develop criteria, review cases where clinical judgment is necessary for full evaluation and to legitimate the work of the non-professional, it is especially appropriate that mental health centers which rely heavily on non-professionals to perform clinical tasks under professional guidance should also use non-professionals in the review process.

THE ADEQUACY OF A THREE-LEVEL REVIEW PROCESS

Prior to the creation of utilization review committees at the centers participating in the PURE Project, review of a particular case would most often be prompted by an inquiry from an insurance company to the medical records department or by a patient's complaint. The chart would then be sent to a senior clinician for review. Rarely did he have available to him any preestablished criteria agreed upon as appropriate for his center.

In order to evaluate whether the checklist approach was as good as this more traditional method of case review, a controlled comparison of the three level review process with other methods for auditing psychiatric records was undertaken.[3] The experimental design called for a comparison of results obtained by employing three different methods to review the same charts. The first of the three methods compared was the open-ended approach (the most traditional). Charts were sent directly to expert clinicians with a request for review and brief instructions to focus on appraising the evaluation and diagnosis of the patient, the disposition, the treatment and the follow-up. The questions were general, but clinicians were encouraged to comment as specifically as possible. The second method was the three-level approach described in this chapter. The expertise of the clinical consultant was used only when violations of checklist criteria were identified. The third method, called the structured clinical questionnaire approach, asked clinicians to answer all 47 specific questions which would be asked in the three-level review if violations of the checklist criteria occurred in all possible situations.

Twenty-seven charts were reviewed three times using each of the three methods. We were interested in the following questions:

1. Does the traditional open-ended approach furnish more specific comments about patient care than either the chart review checklist method or the structured questionnaire method?
2. Do the methods differ in terms of the assessment of the adequacy of care given to patients and of the documentation in the record?
3. Can the time of clinical reviewers be saved by the use of non-clinical research assistants?

We found that the three-level method focused on the majority of issues raised by the traditional open-ended approach to chart review, while the structured questionnaire failed to do so.

To further test the adequacy of the three-level review, three scales were developed to compare the three different approaches. One scale measured the general adequacy of care, the second the adequacy of recording and the third overall adequacy. Analysis of variance was employed to determine whether the methods differed in terms of the assessment of general adequacy as well as of patient care and recording. The results of these analyses indicated that there were no significant differences due to the method of review, the category of the chart or to the interaction of both. The three level method which uses non-clinician research assistants, yielded similar scores for assessed adequacy of charts and overall adequacy of clinical care afforded to patients; adequacy of documentation fell somewhere between satisfactory and excellent.

We were unable to document a savings in clinicians' time because the clinical consultants had been asked to make global assessments of each chart requiring that they read each chart in its entirety. Had they only focused their attention on violations of criteria it is quite probable that there would have indeed been marked savings in clinical consultant time. Thus our data indicate that it is possible the experimental study of a quality control system—utilization review—in a community health center. Our data indicate that chart review can be made more rational and less expensive by introducing a multistage review process which makes use of non-clinical personnel to perform some stages of the review process using preestablished criteria of appropriate care. Such a checklist is as reliable as more traditional methods and potentially more efficient than looser, less structured forms of peer review.

SUMMARY AND CONCLUSIONS

In this chapter we have focused upon a three-level, multistage review process that makes use of non-clinicians to help assess the adequacy of care with the aid of a chart review checklist. This checklist includes preestablished criteria of quality care appropriate for the specific mental health center in which it is operating, measurement scales which can be used both as criteria and as direct measures of quality, and indexes which can be used as selection mechanisms as well as criteria. In both the preceding and the present chapters the problems of establishing validity and reliability and minimizing biases have been addressed. It seems that on an experimental basis the current checklist is as useful as more traditional methods and potentially more valuable in that it saves clinician time. Further, the checklist has the potential for being converted to a computerized system which could work in the framework of already existing systems, such as the Multi-State Information System, or in problem oriented record systems which are also in the process of being computerized.

To our knowledge, there are no examples of case review using pre-established criteria of care in psychiatry; however, there are other examples of individual case review formats reported in the literature.

Newman, et. al.[4] at the American Psychiatric Association Convention in Hawaii, 1973, reported on a utilization review method developed at the Peninsula Hospital Mental Health Center in California. In the face of a financial pinch, the mental health center staff decided to limit outpatient visits to a maximum of six, unless the clinician could justify to the utilization review committee the need for prolonged treatment. Six visits were felt adequate for good diagnostic evaluation and crisis intervention. The model being used is a variation of the case conference with the therapist presenting his work to his colleagues. Unfortunately, there appear to be no recorded criteria which emerged from these conferences, but rather an impression that they function to encourage professionals with a bias toward one-to-one psychotherapy to be more open to other modalities of treatment. Thus, over a period of two years medication maintenance programs were organized and accepted. There was also increasing acceptance of group therapy for patients described as needing more change than could be accomplished in six visits.

Meldmon et. al.[5] at a center in Illinois sent out questionnaires three months after discharge to a sample of patients' families asking about the care received and the current status of the problems which had brought them to seek help. From studies of patient's function and family's satisfaction, certain clinicians were identified as less effective than others. For example, one clinician had a 43 percent dropout rate versus a ten percent to fifteen percent average for all clinicians. It was felt that care would improve if this clinician's performance improved. Thus, the focus of utilization review shifted from the deviant patient to the deviant therapist.

The work of the PURE Project in collaboration with the participating community mental health centers shows that—

1. Standards can be developed in the form of measurement scales, indexes, and preestablished criteria of quality care.
2. Formats can be devised to apply these standards.
3. The standards and the formats for their use can be subject to scientific scrutiny as to their reliability, validity and effectiveness.
4. The development of such standards and the testing of formats is an arduous, time consuming and expensive process. Once developed, however, the use of standards and formats such as the multistage chart review checklist can reduce the amount of effort necessary to perform worthwhile utilization review and patient care evaluation.

Chapter Seven

Selection of Cases for Individual Review

Lee D. Brauer

INTRODUCTION

The advent of legislation of PSROs in the field of medicine has stimulated a new
look at the theory and application of review procedures themselves. The goals of
review are to insure high quality of medical care, efficient delivery of medical
services and also to provide some opportunity for clinical research to delineate
new areas of medical need. The review process involves examination of examples
of desirable or undesirable clinical practice, a sizable task requiring much honest
concern and many man hours of effort. For the review task to be practical,
efficacious and economical, the review procedures themselves must be sensitive,
reliable and efficient. This section will address methods of selecting cases for
review by which the review process itself can be made to yield higher payoff.
Payoff in this sense means more case instances likely to deviate from norms of
care than in a random sample of cases. Without effective methods of selecting
cases for review, the members of a utilization review committee would find the
task unrewarding and the goal of raising standards of care immeasurably more
difficult.

The task of selecting charts for review is a two step procedure. First
one establishes norms for clinical care and then one chooses cases which deviate
from these norms. In order to establish norms for a given dependent variable, a
total population is divided into homogeneous subgroups. For example, while a
normal length of stay in an inpatient service might be fifteen days for the total
population, it is often found that the stay for character disorders is five days, for
neurotic patients ten days and for psychotic patients twenty-three days. This
finding implies that any review of length of stay for this population should
include consideration of diagnosis.

The task of identifying such groups is not trivial. One early approach used in Western Pennsylvania at the Blue Cross of Western Pennsylvania Research Department [1] has been the Automatic Interaction Detection (AID) Program. In this procedure, data about the population are fed into a computer and a dependent variable is specified, such as length of stay. The AID program then automatically subdivides the population, using a statistical procedure which sequentially forms groups and maximally reduces the sum of the variance around the means of the groups formed. This program is fully automated; the groups are formed upon only statistical consideration, and no attempt is made to reconcile them with clinical groupings.

At Yale, researchers working on the same problem and using medical charts and a data base consisting of a brief abstract of all patients in Connecticut hospitals [2] tried a similar approach but found that the groups formed by the fully automated approach were not satisfactory because they often deviated far from clinical comprehensibility. They state "the program was too automatic and often there was no justification available to explain why the computer established certain groups."[2] As a result, the Yale researchers developed AUTOGRP,[4] an interactive computer system, consisting of a set of computer programs to display data and form groups, a data base and a clinical operator. The clinical operator's role was at *each step* of the grouping process, to ascertain the clinical meaningfulness of the results, and to *direct* further evaluation of the data. The operator, rather than the program, defined the groups. While he would usually rely heavily on the results from the statistical display, he could differ when he saw fit. The implementation of this system at Yale–New Haven Hospital (YNHH) was called the Basic Utilization Review Project (BURP), directed by Donald C. Riedel who was also appointed Chairman of the Patient Care Studies Committee of YNHH.

When the question then arose as to whether similar techniques would work in psychiatry, the Psychiatric Utilization Review and Evaluation (PURE) Project attempted an answer. With particular respect to selection mechanisms, the project identified three goals, of which the first was to demonstrate the practicability, utility, economy and efficiency of selecting charts for utilization review and patient care evaluation. The second was to delineate selection mechanisms for case review that would work in several different institutions, some of which would work within given institutions or services. It was expected that some mechanisms could be used directly with no modifications while others would require the specification of parameters unique to a given institution or service. Finally, the project undertook to develop techniques for elaborating and testing such mechanisms. In some instances they would be available for "export;" in others, the techniques would permit institutions which wished to develop their own standards to have some information about how to accomplish this task. The project fulfilled all three goals. The remainder of this chapter is a report on the results.

AN OVERVIEW OF METHODS FOR SELECTING
CASES FOR REVIEW

In order to understand the utility of selection mechanisms, it is necessary to consider a scheme of the review process itself. Elements of the process are discussed in much greater detail in other chapters, but this summary is presented here to highlight where selection may be useful.

Case review is only one component of program evaluation or patient care evaluation. Other components may include pattern-of-care analysis (e.g., are all social classes given opportunity for treatment?) or outcome analysis (did psychotic patients return to the community or were they hospitalized on a chronic service?). Case review is a process by which an individual case (usually an individual treatment episode) is examined to insure that proper and efficient diagnosis and treatment were rendered. A given case is usually reviewed by one or two reviewers, the results presented to a committee for consideration and action. Ideally, all cases would be reviewed and selection would not be necessary. However, the review process itself is expensive. A checklist review by a paramedical reviewer or a clinical review by a clinician each take approximately 30 or 40 minutes. Only a few wealthy institutions with small caseloads can routinely review their entire population.

A general scheme for review using case selection is shown in figure 7–1. The review is accomplished in three stages. The first stage is a check for completeness. Requirements will vary over the course of treatment. A complete record at discharge usually will include an admission note, mental status, diagnosis, progress notes, assessment of condition at time of discharge and disposition. While such a check is desirable for all charts when a case is closed, selection during the course of treatment is possible. For instance, does the chart have an admission diagnosis recorded within two weeks of admission?

Charts may then be selected for review by selection mechanisms. In the scheme listed, all charts selected will be reviewed by a checklist, using fixed criteria for quality of care. The development and application of a checklist for assessment of care is described extensively in chapter 5. This stage of review is often accomplished using paramedical personnel. In stage 3, all charts with some fault on a checklist are sent to a clinician reviewer who uses his judgment to decide if further attention is warranted.

In the scheme described, all charts seen by a clinician have been found lacking by a checklist. Other schemes are possible. Figure 7–2 shows some alternative schemes. With respect to completeness, all three options were considered. Option B is to review all charts for completeness, which is recommended wherever possible. If not possible, some sizable random sample might be checked. It is sometimes feasible (option C) to use some items as flags for an incomplete record. For instance, a missing discharge diagnosis after the discharge might indicate other deficiencies. At times recordkeeping standards of wards may differ,

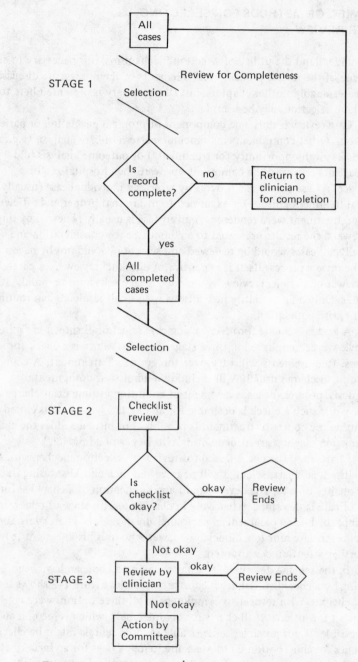

Figure 7–1. General Review Scheme Using Selection

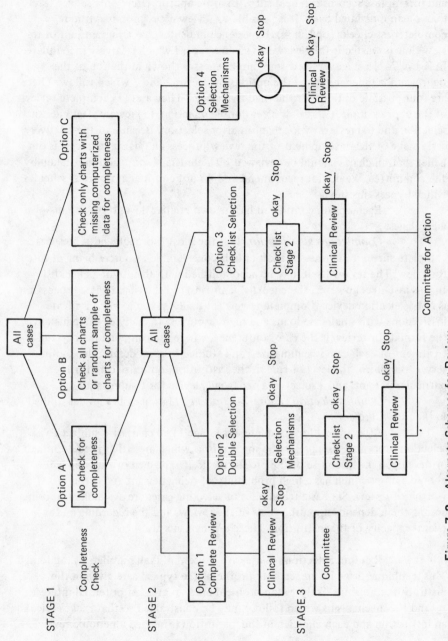

Figure 7-2. Alternate Schemes for Review

and incomplete records can be dealt with more appropriately on a service level than on an individual basis. It is possible to review cases entirely without completeness checks (option A). Experience indicates that a fair amount of review time is wasted if the reviewer is given a record which is largely incomplete. In figure 7-2, a stage 1 review for completeness is shown at the top of the figure, and is independent of the options for stages 2 and 3 which follow. There are four possible options for the final two stages. They are: (1) complete review of the entire sample, (2) review after double selection, (3) review after checklist selection and (4) review by mechanism after selection. Because of the relatively early stage of the development of the review process and its standards, it is our belief that all charts should be reviewed by a clinician before action is taken by the committee. We do not recommend and do not consider as options, schemes which bypass this step.

Each option considered has its own relative advantages and disadvantages.

Complete Review (option 1) is the most thorough and represents a complete survey of all cases seen; it entails considerable resources being devoted to review. The review itself may be accomplished with the use of a checklist. In this instance, however, the checklist is intrinsic to the final review process and is not a selection device. Complete review is usually possible only in private institutions with small case loads and high resources. In many of these instances, the format for review is the case conference, where the complete history and treatment of each case is summarized and studied in great detail. The conference serves to monitor the level of care in the institution, optimize care for the particular patient, and also act as a pedagogic device for training staff.

Double Selection (figure 7-2 option 2) has been the model studied in the PURE Project.

After review for completeness (stage 1) all charts are subject to a selection procedure using selection mechanisms which are either predetermined or developed in the course of the procedure itself. The goal of this step is to choose a chart which has a high probability of being deviant and is therefore worthy of review. Six basic techniques of selecting cases are available. Choosing among them depends upon the goals of the review, and the recording and retrieval capacity of the institution. These mechanisms are:

Random Selection: Cases are chosen in small numbers at random. This technique provides an accurate profile of the typical care given in the institution, but is not likely to tap problem areas or areas of potential interest. It (and the mechanisms which follow) may be constrained so that each service in an institution and each clinician in the institution is insured a periodic review.

Missing Information: Charts where information is missing or late are often worthy of review. Occasionally a missing diagnosis may serve as a flag to an entirely blank record. A consistently high percentage of records with missing information from a particular service may indicate a pattern of care caused by clinical overload of personnel or bad morale.

Selection on the Basis of Problems Felt Worthy of Review: At times there will be a need to review charts in relation to special problems noted within a given facility. For example, a utilization review committee might elect to focus on a known problem such as a sudden increase in adolescents signing out against medical advice. Cases selected for review would all be illustrative of the problem under study. One mental health center elected to review four suicide attempts occurring on one treatment unit in a two-week period. The review was able to identify particular staff conflicts which had led to the ward disruption.

Exceptional Cases Defined by Deviation from Norms: This mechanism is grounded on normative criteria for the quality of care. For instance, a particular facility may have established a criterion that all patients with the diagnosis of schizophrenia should receive phenothiazines. The utilization review committee could then request from treatment units or clinicians a list of schizophrenic patients who are not receiving phenothiazines. These cases would then be subject to a more detailed review.

Aberrant Care Identified by Analysis of the Pattern of Care: In this system, the selection of a chart for review is indicated when it violates one or more statistical norms established through the review of patterns of care in a specific institution. For instance, cases could be selected in which the pattern of care (e.g., duration or type of treatment) varies in either direction from the norm for a patient in a given diagnostic category on a given service. If examination of the psychiatric records indicate that such care does indeed frequently prove to be inappropriate, meaningful cutoff points can then be established. These cutoff points would enclose the range of probably good care; variations beyond these points would have a high probability of being inappropriate. A manual selection procedure or computer program which automatically flags deviant cases of patient care can report a series of such cases on a regular basis to the utilization review committee.

Selection on the Basis of Length of Stay or Source of Payment: Here the selection of cases for review is generally governed by requirements of third-party carriers and the federal government concerning payment for services rendered. At times a facility will need to justify certain treatment interventions and durations of stay. Once criteria related to extended duration have been established, this method of selecting case review can become a routine process.

The above techniques for selecting charts may be used in combination with one another. For instance, all charts may be checked for missing data at specified intervals, and other charts selected by such standards as length of stay or condition on discharge. In addition when particular problems exist, charts may be selected at that time for those specific reasons.

One requirement of the selection procedure is that the total number of charts selected be no greater than can be examined by the checklist. When the number is greater, the reviewer may arbitrarily select a subsample of charts chosen either according to interest, at random, or to fulfill an ancillary review requirement such as periodic review of a particular service or clinician.

Charts selected are then reviewed by a checklist (stage 2). The checklist is a thorough review of all aspects of a record according to predetermined criteria for quality of care. The checklist may have separate sections which apply only to particular classes of cases, (e.g., adolescents, suicidal patients, schizophrenics). Although at this point the checklist is filled out by hand by paramedical personnel, ultimately it may be computerized and filled in by machine. This would require both the programming of the checklist, which is relatively simple, and the computer collection of all data required to answer the questions, which is a more difficult task, in fact if not in principle. The use and development of checklists are described more thoroughly in chapter 6.

No chart which is adequate by checklist standards is assumed to need clinical review. However, only charts selected by both "mechanism" and checklist are given to a clinician for a clinical impression. This impression is not based on predetermined criteria, but rather on clinical assessment of the treatment involved.

A chart may fail for reasons not directly related to the mechanism that selected it. It is perfectly conceivable that a chart selected for review because of excessive length of stay will fail the checklist because medications required for the condition were not administered and fail the clinical reviewer because diagnosis was inadequately established or discharge plans were not discussed with the family. The indexes for selection are a complexly determined variable, and the procedure is often statistical-empirical rather than clinical-logical. That a length of stay was long for a given patient compared to similar patients does not necessarily imply bad care, but it is the result of bad care in a significant enough number of instances to be associated with violation of other clinical norms. Each step of the review procedure adds information. The checklist serves initially as a selection procedure and later as an adjunct to the review procedure. Cases which pass are not reviewed by a clinician. When cases do not pass, the reasons for selection and the checklist may be sent to the clinician as an initial basis for his review.

To summarize briefly, in this prototype procedure, charts are—

1. checked for completeness,
2. selected by mechanisms,
3. reviewed by checklists,

4. reviewed by clinicians, and
5. voted on by the committee.

Variants of this procedure involve the omission of one significant step. In checklist selection (option 3) no selection procedure is used. Since mechanisms are seldom available or resources adequate to review all charts by a checklist procedure (for most institutions this is prohibitively expensive), a random sample is usually taken. This is, to be sure, a selection procedure; but it is not designed to enhance the probability that charts will be deviant. In fact, it is more likely to provide the committee with a profile of typical care in the institution. While this has the advantage of not requiring retrievable information for use in selection (i.e., no coded abstracts or computerized records), it results in reviews with a lower payoff and possible loss of interest in their work on the part of the committee.

In institutions where the likelihood of deviance is high, selection may not be needed, for any case chosen at random will be productive and random selection is feasible.

Mechanism selection (option 4) does not require the use of a checklist *as a selection mechanism*. Rather, charts are fed directly to a clinical reviewer who may or may not use predetermined criteria. When a computer system and clinicians are available, this option has the advantage of permitting the institution of a new review process with no delay for evaluation or development of a checklist.

In institutions where charts selected by mechanism are highly likely to be selected also by a checklist, the checklist ceases to be an important factor in selection, but remains important as an adjunct to the final clinical review process.

Most institutions undertaking review have found criteria development (checklist development) a necessary preliminary step in clarifying their comprehension of the review process and specifying their goals in the institutional setting.

RESULTS OF SELECTING CASES FOR REVIEW

A study of selection mechanisms was undertaken at four participating institutions. Two did sufficient work for results to emerge. A third institution developed a checklist and procedures but did not use computer selection of records. The fourth selected all charts at random in order to obtain a profile.

In the two institutions that did test selection mechanisms, each used the three stage review procedure described in the previous section. One of the institutions tested charts selected by computer-derived mechanisms against a comparable random sample. The other tested charts selected by computer-derived mechanisms against a sample of charts selected according to the interests of its committee members and standards suggested by them on an a priori basis. (Fig. 7–3)

In both instances, charts selected were evaluated by a checklist, used as a *secondary selector*, and a clinician reviewed only charts that failed to pass the checklist. There was no test of checklist selection against mechanism selection and the clinicians reviewed no random sample of charts, so there was no specific test at the level of third stage review of selected versus unselected charts.

Table 7–1 presents the results of the checklist test (stage 2) of selected versus unselected charts. It is clearly seen that there is a statistically significant enhancement of the probability that a selected chart warrants review. Only ten of 116 selected charts did not warrant clinical review. Also, significant in its own

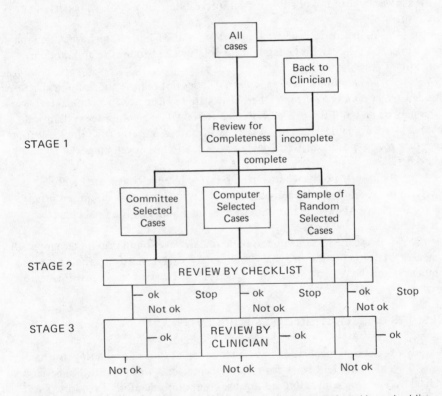

N.B. All cases reviewed by clinician had been reviewed by a checklist first and found positive.

Clinicians reviewed no cases not first found deficient at Stage 2 (Checklist Review).

Figure 7–3. Experimental Design for Evaluating Results of Case Selection

Table 7-1. Checklist Test: Mechanism Selected vs. Random (stage 2)

	Needs More Review +	*No Further Review* −	
Mechanism	106	10	116
Random	86	21	107
Total	192	31	223

$X^2 = 5.63$

$p < 0.02$

Eighty-six percent of all charts need more review

right, is the finding that only 21 of 107 randomly selected charts did not need review. The results may be summarized as follows:

1. Most records in the sample, selected or unselected, warrant review (86 percent).
2. Selected charts are significantly more likely to warrant review.

Table 7-2 shows that there is no statistically significant difference at the level of clinical review (stage 3) between charts selected by checklist and mechanism compared to checklist only. These results indicate that where a checklist could be used on all charts, there would be no additional benefit in preliminary computer selection. However, the previous results clearly show that computer preselection will increase the efficiency of a three stage review procedure, when all charts are not reviewed by checklists.

Tables 7-3 and 7-4 indicate that there are no significant differences between results obtained from mechanisms and those suggested by a committee or a computer. It speaks well for both. A center without computer resources can meaningfully select charts using a priori criteria, and a center with computer resources may elect to have the procedure done automatically.

Table 7-2. Clinical Review (stage 3): Checklist and Mechanisms vs. Checklist Only

	Refer to Committee +	*Okay* −	
Checklist and Mechanisms	84	22	106
Checklist only	66	20	86
Total	150	42	192

$X^2 = 0.1738$

$p > 5$ not significant

Seventy-eight percent of all charts refer to committee.

Table 7-3. Checklist Test: Computer Selection vs. Committee Selection (stage 2).

	Needs Review +	Does Not Need Review −	
Computer	44	57	101
Committee	41	63	104
Total	85	120	205

$X^2 = .036$

$p > .5$

Forty-one percent of all charts need review.

A comparison of tables 7–1 against 7–3 or 7–2 against 7–4 will indicate that at both stage 2 and stage 3 levels, in one center a much higher percentage of charts warrant review. Several questions remain unanswered. It is not possible to say whether this is a result of differing levels of care or of more stringent criteria in the checklist and clinical review. One would want to know how mechanism-selected cases compare with randomly selected cases at third level review, with no preselection by checklist. In tables 7–3 and 7–4, a random sample would be useful to test for enhanced results due to selection. However, each case reviewed required from one and one-half to three hours of clinical, paramedical and committee time. The test of the selection mechanism was not the only goal of the study, for the utility of the criteria concept and of review itself were major issues. The resources available to the study and the participating institutions precluded those tests at that time.

The result that selection of charts either clinically or statistically deviant enhance the efficiency of the review process is important but not unexpected. A more surprising result is that a large percentage of charts requires review. The question not answered by the simple index of the study is about the

Table 7-4. Clinical Review: Computer and Checklist vs. Committee and Checklist

	Refer to Committee +	Okay −	
Computer and Checklist	20	9	29
Committee and Checklist	18	14	32
Total	38	23	61

$X^2 = 1.05$

$p > .3$

Sixty-two percent of all charts refer to committee.

level and degree of the deviance uncovered. The high percentage of charts requiring review could represent either a marked deficiency in the quality of care or simply an indication that the review procedure is a quite sensitive instrument and that something can be learned from almost any case. The answer to this question is not provided in the methodology of this part of the study, but can be approximated by the results of the review procedures and the attitudes of the reviewers toward these results reported in chapter 6.

The focus for the remainder of this chapter will shift to the techniques for development of the selection mechanisms themselves.

SELECTION MECHANISMS FOR CASE REVIEW IN PSYCHIATRY

A selection mechanism is a rule for choosing a chart to review. Pragmatic considerations have strongly influenced the development of such mechanisms. These considerations are based largely on retrievability of information. For example, one might wish to select charts when there is a marked psychosocial discord between the clinician and the patient. These might include countertransference reactions, failure of empathy, or such cultural dissimilarity that prejudices in either clinician or patient cannot be perceived or overcome. However, information at this level of abstraction is usually not recorded directly and is almost never recorded on computerized forms. Although some simplistic indexes based on age, race or sex differences between clinician and patient might approximate this type of factor, even that represents a level of sophistication beyond that attained at the present time. It is yet only a clinical presumption that these indexes and factors would be more germane than those which can more readily be measured. The superiority of mechanisms derived from information at a higher level of abstraction remains a presumption.

We undertook to develop selection mechanisms using information that was precoded and retrievable by computers. During the course of this study, the quantity and quality of such information has been remarkably enhanced. At the beginning of our work, only information about sociodemographic factors, total length of stay, rudimentary treatment and discharge was available. Work recently completed or about to be completed at the time of this writing, has added detailed information about symptomatology, presenting problems, course of treatment, length of stay on each ward, type of clinical intervention and identity of the primary clinician. Some of the new data resulted from the addition of new forms to the system, and the rest from special programs designed to retrieve, on a routine basis, information stored in the system. An additional new type of input is based on mathematically derived scales which condense large amounts of information into a few variables. Factor analysis was used to derive these scales.

Our experience has repeatedly indicated that selection is possible with some retrieval capability at some level of sophistication and also that development of the system for retrieval is an ongoing part of the process of review. At any state of development there is always a next step that seems desirable. The value and expense of such development must be balanced against the potential value of its application to other aspects of the process.

The mechanisms we derived and used are included in appendix 7–A. Some mechanisms require more information than others. Some mechanisms apply across institutions and others apply only within a specific institution. Some require only retrieval capacity while others require the ability to calculate indexes (e.g., average and standard deviation (S.D.), length of stay). Finally, others require full interactive capability between a clinician and a data system in order to identify relevant parameters and ancillary statistical capability for use as a guide to relevant variables or in development of scales.

Accordingly, we have organized the mechanisms we have used in order of increasing complexity and decreasing generality. Mechanisms are presented in the three lists:

1. *Universal* applies across institutions.
2. *Institution specific* applies with a particular institution and across time.
3. *Run specific* applies for a particular institution and a particular time.

Each list is divided into two sections: the first requires only recording and retrieval of the specific variables used; the second requires some statistical capability to perform calculations on specific variables such as the standard deviation of a length of stay of a specified group of patients.

The universal mechanisms are intended to be used as specific rules for selecting charts for review. Any center, by perusing the list, may find mechanisms which focus on issues relevant to their goals that can be used directly. A center desiring to develop its own selection procedure may find ideas about the relevant variables and types of rules which have been used. Most mechanisms are very specific and produce few, if any, charts in most instances. They are primarily designed for large data sets with full retrieval capability. There are over 100 mechanisms specified; many of them are in general form and represent a large number of mechanisms condensed into a single statement (*see* appendix 7–A, Specification of Mechanisms in a Tree Form). Far more mechanisms have been developed than have been tested. The test performed was an aggregate—charts were selected by one or more of the mechanisms on these lists or at random. We cannot specify which proved most fruitful. It will take experience far beyond the intended scope of this study to discriminate among the mechanisms in detail.

It is occasionally necessary to have extensive information available to ask relevant questions (e.g., appendix 7–A, A.1.). To review inpatient care it was necessary to have information on symptoms, diagnosis, duration of condition and age. When such information was present, sizable groups with high probability (0.93) or low probability (.02) of an inpatient treatment could be determined.

There is considerable importance to the result that review mechanisms derived by clinicians from a particular institution not using statistical information performed as well as mechanisms derived by a clinician relatively unfamiliar with the institution but using statistical techniques. Clinicians in an institution, especially if they have some access to rudimentary data processing, should be able to develop effective mechanisms by combining some of the specific mechanisms we suggest with ones they feel are relevant, where particular parameters (such as average length of stay for a particular condition) are available as a guide.

The next section will deal with the techniques for developing the selection mechanisms. An attempt will be made to show both the usefulness of standard analytic procedures and also the additional benefit which occurs for access to more advanced statistical systems. AUTOGRP, a statistical system designed specifically for the purpose of selecting charts for review, will be discussed in its current and future forms.

TECHNIQUES FOR DEVELOPING
SELECTION MECHANISMS

Of first consideration in developing a set of mechanism for selecting charts to review is the availability of information. The record must contain the information called for in the mechanism and this information must also be retrievable with relative facility.

Most institutions rely on handwritten records with typed summaries, with varying degrees of adequacy, quality and completeness. Hypothetically, if one wished to review geriatric alcoholics, it would be necessary to read in the record room all charts until by chance a sufficient sample was obtained. This might take ten or fifteen minutes a chart and be for all practical purposes inefficient and prohibitive, for it would be repeatedly required. Some alternative is needed. It might be possible to work closely with the staff of the treating units to obtain lists of patients who fit certain criteria, e.g., patients discharged against advice, those who attempt suicide, schizophrenics not given phenothiazines or patients with multiple admissions.

One inexpensive retrieval system is a tab-card abstract. A few basic variables can be coded on these cards, usually by bending or hand punching a tab. They may be initiated at the time of admission and completed upon discharge. These tab cards contain certain rudimentary but vital information on admission, including age, sex, ethnicity, ward of admission, number of previous hospitalizations, diagnosis and primary clinician. On discharge, one card would indicate the type of discharge, some coded appraisal of outcome and length of stay. Such a relatively simple system contains much of the pertinent information used for retrieval in larger systems and is probably adequate for smaller centers' needs. For a center with handwritten records, it provides an intermediate alternative to an expensive computer system. Preparing an abstracted card requires only a few minutes at admission, a few more minutes at discharge. Retrieval time is minimal. The chart is read only once to prepare the abstract.

Computer techniques currently in use require precoded forms which contain information about sociodemographic factors, diagnosis, symptoms, history, treatment and outcome. The richer the data base, the more sophisticated and refined are the selection possibilities. Meaningful selection is possible even if the data base includes only ward, type of treatment and length of stay. However, enhanced selection is possible if one can relate information such as symptoms and diagnosis to the patient's treatment.

Precoded information may reflect the patient's problem only indirectly. For example, the isolated schizophrenic is more likely to require review than one with social contacts (a job or family). In most cases, social isolation will not be a precoded category, forcing one to use a category such as "lives alone" in selecting cases for review. Needless to say, the fact that a schizophrenic lives alone does not necessarily mean he is socially isolated but it is more likely to be correlated with isolation than chance selection. As precoded forms are developed further, more relevant parameters may be added. At the present time, however, the advantages of precoded information for selecting charts for review outweigh the disadvantages, because techniques are not yet commonly available to automatically code, categorize and process data written in plain English. For instance, a mental health center in an inner city might very well be concerned with the review of cases involving black adolescents who are parents, drug addicted, depressed, on welfare and who have quit treatment. The retrieval of information with that degree of specificity requires a fairly complete retrieval procedure. With greater retrieval sophistication, patients sixty-five or older whose recorded diagnosis does not reflect their alcoholic symptomatology could be selected as a group of special interest to geriatric service. The study of this group would require the presence of problem appraisal data, in addition to more routine sociodemographic and diagnostic information.

Utility of a computer system is closely related to the processing capacity of the system and the quality of the information in the data base. A more sophisticated retrieval system enables a center to adopt a more elaborate review procedure. In general, all systems have a sorting capacity that can list patients who meet specified criteria; almost all systems possess some ability to generate routine reports containing averages and tables. More sophisticated systems provide, with varying degrees of ease, flexibility and capacity, statistical techniques to identify interrelationships among the variables stored in a system. In turn, these relationships elucidate norms of practice. In a center with resources for only retrieval and tabulation, norms for selection of charts may be established a priori or derived in proximate fashion from tabular output. For instance, charts indicating multiple admissions within a single year, worsening of condition at the time of discharge or leaving against medical advice may require review. However, determination of length of stay as a function of diagnosis and type of treatment may require statistical capability that exceeds the resources of most mental health centers. Depending upon the statistical capacity of the system and the interest and sophistication of the user, more-or-less precise and specific selection mechanisms may be specified.

Alternatives exist for institutions with minimal statistical capacity to tailor mechanisms to their own standards and resources. For example, many community mental health centers treat situational crisis reactions in special units with definite limits on length of stay. A review of patients whose stay exceeds this institutional limit may be of interest. An institution with a large outpatient treatment program may consider age a major factor in determining outcome. "Discharged against medical advice" may be uncommon in the geriatric group and, therefore, worthy of review. However, this may be acceptable or even desirable in the population of adolescents. A cross tabulation of outpatients' ages and types of discharge would establish whether this selection mechanism, which has worked in other institutions, would be fruitful in this institution.

Given the existence of a computer system with retrieval capacity, selection mechanisms can be preprogrammed and run at monthly or quarterly intervals. Similarly, routine reports about length of stay, number of patients seen on a service and number of patients and treatment hours for each clinician may be generated. These reports might serve as a means for selecting cases of either underactive or overactive clinicians.

After consideration of the recording, retrieval and processing power of a system, there remains the question of how information is used to generate selection mechanisms. For heuristic purposes, it is easiest to describe this process using the techniques of an interactive statistical reporting system designed specifically for this purpose and then to consider how these results might be approximated using statistical techniques more commonly available.

AUTOGRP [15] is the name given a man-machine interactive computer system consisting of a user, a data base and a computer language, designed to facilitate rapid analysis of complex medical information. The clinical or administrative expertise of the user is combined with sophisticated computer techniques to permit rapid information retrieval and identification of deviant cases. The unique feature of the system is the stepwise interaction of the clinical knowledge of the user with immediate statistical display of information in the data base which permits results of a composite nature not possible through clinical or statistical approaches alone.

Using length of stay as the dependent variable, for example, an entire patient population can be grouped according to combinations of identifiable characteristics such as age, sex, diagnosis, admission problems and ward of admission. Norms for length of stay are developed for particular segments of the population. From these norms cases treated for periods longer or shorter than the average for their defined group are selected for further scrutiny. The hypothesis upon which this type of review is based is that these cases are more likely to represent inappropriate or inefficient instances of care than cases closer to the mean of the distribution for any particular dependent variable. It is, of course, quite likely that some cases of innovative practice will also be selected because they also may depart from expected values.

The Development of the AUTOGRP System

AUTOGRP is used to define interactively the groups used in this process. Other programs currently in use set norms non-interactively from which cases are selected. The heart of the AUTOGRP system contains an algorithm for forming subgroups from an original population.

The user selects a dependent and independent variable and the population to be categorized. The algorithm then performs the following operations:

1. Compute the mean and variance for the entire original population of group.
2. For each category of the independent variable, compute the means of the dependent variable and arrange the categories according to means.
3. Sequentially, split the parent group at every possible point and compute the new mean and variance for each new group.
4. *Define a "break" point for the group where the sum of the variance for each new group is maximally reduced. This uniquely defines two new groups from the original group.*
5. Iterate this procedure (steps 3 and 4) on each new group formed until the total variance reduced by breaking a group is less than a specified proportion (usually one percent) of the total variance of the original group.[4]

The process leads to the formation of new groups which for any categorical variable reduce the variance around the means of the dependent variable. One measure of the strength of the grouping is the percentage of the original variance reduced by forming the new groups. These groups were presented to the clinical operator who would modify them, use them, or disregard them on the basis of clinical knowledge. The clinical operator defined all groups. He also controlled the search strategy and could use his knowledge to test expected relationships in areas of high payoff.

The AUTOGRP control language as it exists now has as its essential component parts:

1. An algorithmic procedure for grouping data according to similarity of distribution of some dependent variable for both continuous and categorical independent variables,
2. A control language which could be learned by an unsophisticated user whose contribution to the system would be clinical knowledge,
3. A rapid display of the data to the user and rapid statistical operations on the data,
4. A method of storing and recalling groups formed, along designated characteristics.

AUTOGRP was the tool used throughout the past two years of this project to develop mechanisms for review.

Some examples may serve to clarify its use and show the scheme for developing other mechanisms: example 1 (see figure 7-4) the population chosen was all patients admitted after January 1972, who were already discharged. A total of 3193 were seen with an average length of stay on ward of admission of 41.3 and a standard deviation of 57.6.

For 95 percent confidence, no lower limit is possible and an upper limit is 157.0 days, (mean + 2 Standard Deviations).

A search of likely variables at point **B** shows 28.2 percent of the variance is accounted for by the ward the person was admitted to. This has been the most consistent finding in surveying length of stay data—time spent is largely determined by ward policy. A new variable, **Y**, value 1 if transferred, 0 if not, is created at point **C** to test the hypothesis that people transferred to a different ward have shorter length of stay on the admission ward and longer total length of stay in the institution. Point **D** shows an admission stay is 20.7, average 29.4 standard deviation with transfer. Without transfer, admission stay is 51.6, standard deviation is 65.1. Point **E** shows total length of stay is increased from 52 days to 108 days if there is a transfer during treatment.

However, the most powerful variable was ward of admission. The AUTOGRP algorithm suggests four groups of wards at point **F**. They are named SHORT, MEDIUM, LONG AND VERY LONG, and these four groups are chosen as the first subdivision in the population. While still containing considerable unresolved variance, nonetheless, it is seen the mean LOS now ranges from 15.6 days to 137.8 for these groups.

These groups are repeatedly surveyed and subdivided. As can be seen by point **G**, three of the four groups were split, one twice and the others once. The MEAN LENGTH OF STAY on the admission ward ranges from 3.7 MEAN 3.28 STANDARD DEVIATION—group ADPD—to 166.15 MEAN 107.3 STANDARD DEVIATION—Group MSNG.

The variables which proved important in forming the tree are shown in figure 7-5. This finding is typical of the institution surveyed. In other ex-

Figure 7-4. Example of AUTOGRP Session to Partition Variance for Length of Stay

---

==>> MAKE LOSADM DEP

==>> STATISTICS DIS   A
    3193   41.3   57.6

==>> SEARCH DIS USING ADX WDADM AGE SEX EDUC INCOME
$$$$$

NAME	TSS	REDUCTION		B
ADX	9916843.00	6.4%		
WDADM	7604313.00	28.2%		
AGE	9777088.00	7.7%	CONTIGUOUS	
SEX	10591399.00	.0%		
EDUC	10266001.00	3.1%		
INCOME	10443054.00	1.4%		

***ORIGINAL TSS = 10591399.00

==>> CREATE Y FROM DATA W . E "WDMR1 > 0"   C
$$Y   CREATED

==>> BREAK Y OF DIS   D
2 CELLS. TSS   = 10591399.00
2 GROUPS. TSS = 9906707.00 94%

FROM	TO	SIZE	MEAN	S.D.	SUM. SQ	
1	1	1073	20.68	29.41	928310.25	A
2	2	2120	51.58	65.08	8978397.00	A

==>> DISPLAY Y OF DIS   E
$2 CELLS.

CT	NUM	MEAN TOTLOS	S.D. TOTLOS	Y
1	2120	52.69	65.09	0
2	1073	107.79	90.61	1

==>> CLASSIFY WDADM OF DIS   F
24 CELLS. TSS   = 10591399.00
4 GROUPS. TSS = 7604313.00   72%

********		902	15.54	27.67	696577.75	BA
1	111	348	4.3			
2	210	119	16.4			
3	220	1	20.0			
4	500	431	24.3			
5	132	2	25.5			
6	501	1	28.0			
********		1872	38.45	48.15	4340842.00	EBA
7	520	5	32.6			
8	634	1	35.0			
9	200	384	37.7			
10	100	1482	38.7			
********		183	72.28	66.16	800972.87	EBA
11	230	9	55.7			
12	130	6	63.0			
13	400	23	66.4			

Figure 7-4 continued

```
14   599       78 70.0
15   530        5 73.2
16   131       38 79.6
17   310       26 81.8

********      236 137.81     86.65    1771922.00 A
18   202    166134.2
19   133     33134.4
20   588     13137.9
21   201     13150.9
22   233      5162.8
. . . etc.
```

==>>SUMMARIZE   ·G

```
SIZE     MEAN      S.D.     SUM.SQ
 164      3.70      3.24       1727  ADPD-----+-VYSHORT---  +-SHORT---+
                                                       ]             ]         ]
 184      4.00      3.03       1692  SCHIZ----+         ]         ]
 554     12.59     33.34     615818            SHRT -------+         ]
 752     22.78     27.79     580600            XFER -------+-MED ----+
                                                       ]         ]
1120     49.38     55.31    3426888            NOXFER ----+         ]
  27     94.37     65.07     114332            DEPDOPG ---+ VYLONG--+
                                                       ]             ]
 146    134.05     75.93     553201            TSDNSCH----+         ]
                                                       ]             ]
  61    166.15    107.30     702360            MSNG -------+         ]
                                                                 ]
 183     72.28     66.16     800973                         LONG----+
```

==>>SHOW BY NOXFER   H

```
  0-   29   363  ***********************************
 30-   59   239  **********************
 60-   89   118  *********
 90-  119    74  ******
120-  149    51  ****
150-  179    41  ***
180-  209    24  **
210-  239    13
240-  269     9
270-  299     1
300-  329     0
330-  359     1
```

amples during the course of the work, it has been possible to account for 45 to 50 percent of the total variance in length of stay. A mathematical characteristic of the algorithm used makes it acceptable for the same variable to account for successive division in a tree, and typically diagnosis and internal transfer most powerfully effect length of stay although nowhere near so powerfully as ward of admission. This is in marked contrast to general medicine, where institutional policy is secondary to the natural course of the disease.

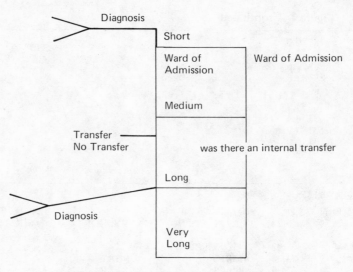

Figure 7–5. Variables Used to Form Tree

At the end of the run, point **G** is a histogram of the large group NOXFER where little further variance could be explained. The shape of the length of stay curve is exponential, and a cutoff is visually assigned at 209 days. Patients who stay longer than that are selected for review. This is a somewhat stricter cutoff than the MEAN = 2 S.D., but yields few patients with greater probability of aberrance. Similarly, one might wish to assign a 10–day cutoff to group ADPD, who are patients seen on a crisis unit, or an 11–day cutoff to those on that unit who have a diagnosis of schizophrenia or alcoholism.

Other dependent variables have proven important in this work. Condition on discharge, simply rated on a 1 to 7 scale, provides a valuable indicator of outcome. In some conditions, improvement may be expected (affective disorders typically improve), in others, it is the exception (personality disorder often leave AMA and with no improvement).

Missing data can be made a dependent variable. Ward patterns or record-keeping are often reflected in surveys of missing data. A "diagnosis undetermined" is used to hide an alcoholic condition or serves as a guide to a patient who presents an unusual problem. This category has repeatedly accounted for considerable variation in type of discharge, length of stay and failure to improve. The variable may be used to specify a case worth reviewing while still in treatment.

Example 1 required only diagnostic and sociodemographic data. Ultimately, all that it needed was diagnostic data and information about the ward of treatment and transfers. Since ward has such a profound effect on length of stay, it was decided to survey assignment to ward of treatment in one institution where problems at the time of admission were recorded. The tree which developed in this survey of inpatient status is presented in figure 7-6. The dependent

Figure 7-6. Example of AUTOGRP Summary Statement Displaying Contribution of Factors in Determining Probability of Hospitalization

==>> SUMMARIZE

SIZE	MEAN	S.D	SUM.SQ
131	.20	.40	21
1745	.03	.18	58
194	.22	.42	33
124	.39	.49	29
624	.20	.40	101
46	.57	.50	11
149	.92	.27	11
603	.53	.50	150

615 ORIGINAL SUMSQ. 415 REMAINING SUMSQ. 32.58% REDUCTION.

```
AGIORI ----+-CHRDX.1----+-CHR------+-NOTPSY
           ]            ]          +----------+
NOAGDO----+              ]                     ]
                         ]                     ]
           CHRDX.2----+  ]                     ]
                      +--+                      ]
           CHRDX.3----+                         ]
                                                ]
                      ACU------+                ]
           GDDX------+-ACUTE---+-PSYCHO----+    ]
           BDDX------+                     +----+
                      CHRONIC ----+
```

variable is the proportion of patients in any group who were hospitalized. Note the groups NOAGDO and BDDX. For NOAGDO, only 3 percent were hospitalized, BDDX, 92 percent. NOAGDO is defined by the following conditions:

1. No hallucinations, delusions, suicidal acts, inappropriate affect, disorientation, withdrawal, agitation.
2. Had illness for duration greater than or equal to one year.
3. Had diagnosis of: no mental disorder, transient situational disturbance, alcoholism, diagnosis deferred, personality disorder.
4. Had no agitation or disorientation.

The specification for BDDX was:

1. Had *at least one* of the symptoms in previous example.
2. Had duration of condition less than one year.
3. Had diagnosis of alcoholism, no mental disorder, diagnosis deferred, personality disorder, affective disorder, schizophrenic/functional psychosis, neurosis, drug dependent. (This excludes organic brain syndrome, transient situational disturbance, and diagnosis deferred.)

For these groups the questions for review are, respectively, "Why was the patient hospitalized?" and "Why wasn't the patient hospitalized?" Similar work was possible for admission to the children's ward or admission to an alcohol unit or in the relationship between alcohol as a symptom in diagnosis, and in assignment to an alcoholism unit for treatment.

It would be clear by this point that the number of questions one might ask is limitless, and considerations of time and institutional interests tended to govern the focus of any particular run. Much of this work was done in anticipation of requests from centers, for the scheduling demanded development of techniques to derive the mechanisms before particular institutions were prepared to use them. Must of the more interesting work has not yet been tested by the committees.

Early experience in developing mechanisms resulted in a marked development of the AUTOGRP system itself. The system's use was seen most clearly as an adjunctive tool to the review committee. It functioned with sufficient rapidity to be available even during the course of a meeting. The AUTOGRP system has undergone the following developmental changes: its storage capacity has been increased to handle such large data sets; some creation of new variables is now possible. Work currently in progress will result in virtually limitless storage capacity.[5] It will be possible to subject variables to algebraic manipulation, permitting the development of scales and creation of new variables. Search procedures will be semiautomatic and the clinical operator will be able to program strategies of search as well as carry them out stepwise.

Other statistical techniques will be integrated into the system, so immediate factor analysis, correlation analysis and multiple regression will be available to locate relevant relationships.

To summarize briefly, AUTOGRP is an interactive computer system which uses an algorithm to suggest homogeneous groups and a clinician to define search strategies and ascertain if the groups mathematically found are clinically meaningful.

How are other techniques relevant to this procedure, and how do they differ from AUTOGRP? AUTOGRP makes no assumptions about linear relationships between a set of dependent and independent variables. It deals with one scaled dependent and one categorical variable. Other techniques usually assume both the variables are continuous (scaled) and look for relationships among them. It is often possible to "dummy" a categorical variable and then apply linear techniques. The dummy variable is assigned the value of 1 if a condition holds true and 0 if it does not. Each category is dealt with as a separate dummy variable, so categorical data can be adapted to linear analysis. Three important techniques warrant brief discussion. Most important is correlation analysis. Correlation analysis provides a measure of association between two continuous variables. If one has a list of symptoms, and wishes to know how they relate, one can intercorrelate them. Figure 7–7 is an example of such a matrix. Note, in the column labeled Delusions, the items which intercorrelate all appeared as relevant in the AUTOGRP example about hospitalization.

A clinician can use such intercorrelations directly to develop a scale score for symptoms related to a treatment or diagnosis and say that if a person scores over a given value on the scale, he should have been hospitalized or his case should be reviewed. For the AUTOGRPer, such a matrix provides a rapid guide to likely important factors and reduces search time considerably.

Correlation coefficient deals with only two variables at a time. Often a number of variables intercorrelate together. Factor analysis is a statistical technique which treats each variable as an independent dimension and sets up an orthogonal axis in an N-dimensional space based on intercorrelations. Items which vary together, called factors, are projected on the same axis, and the factors can be used as new variables often containing the effect of several of the old ones combined. Every patient can be scored on every factor, and these scores are a convenient manner of summarizing with items which are highly correlated.

Figure 7–8 shows the results of a factor analysis of the data used to determine need for hospitalization in the previous example. Note that all items which appeared in the list of symptoms are present on factor 1. This suggests several ways the factor analysis might be used. If one were constructing mechanisms using the AUTOGRP system, the factor analysis would immediately suggest the relevant items to test for construction of a mechanism.

It is also possible to use factor scores to identify cases. Patients with a high score on factor 1 should probably be hospitalized, and those with a low

Figure 7-7.   Correlation Analysis Matrix

	Suspic Persc	Speech Probs	Suicid Acts	Delusions	Agit Hyperac	Anxiety Phob	Hallucinate	Disorn Memry
Delusions	.439							
Hallucinate	.304							
Inapp Affect	.223							
OPeople Prob	.209							
Spch Dis Inc		.215						
Suicid Thgts			.499					
Depres Infer			.241					
Suspic Persc				.439				
Agit Hyperac				.202				
Hallucinate				.464				
Inapp Affect				.248				
Delusions					.202			
Anger Negatv					.266			
Assaultive					.235			
Inapp Affect					.208			
Sleep Problems						.208		
Suspic Persc						.221		
Deprs Infer						.336		
Withdrwl Iso						.255		
OPeople Prob						.221		
Suspic Persc							.304	
Delusions							.464	
Inapp Affect							.225	
Spch Dis Inc								.245
Inapp Affect								.253

Figure 7-8. Results of Factor Analysis

Grandiosity	.325					
Suspic	.641					
Delusions	.705					
Agit Hyperac	.378					
Hallucinate	.586					
Anger Negatv	.323					
Assaultive	.400					
Inapp Affect	.379					
Schizo. Funct. Disord	.614					
Inpatient versus Others	-.466					
Sleep Problems		.590				
Eating Problems		.634				
Job Problems		.551				
Seizure Conv		.327				
Mate Problems		.414				
Alcohol Abuse		.656				
Alcoholism		.539				
Suicid Thgts			.713			
Suicid Acts			.713			
Deprs Affect			.532			
Affective Disorders			.630			
Inpatient versus Others			-.342			
School Problems				.640		
Anti Soc Attitude				.354		
Agit Hyperact				.355		
Anger Negativity				.537		
Assaultive				.365		
Family Problems				.410		
Other People Problems				.399		
Trans Situat Disord				.539		
Narco Drugs					.828	
Drug Dependency					.815	
Speech Problems						.314
Disorn Memory						.588
Inad Intell						.384
Spch Dis Inc						.507
Emotion Lack						.482
Inapp Affect						.479
RTN, LSR IMPR						.459
Dependency						.333
Diagnosis Missing						.307
Mental Retard – OBS						.215
Inpatient versus Others						.356
Anxiety Phob						.510
Depres Infer						.457
Alcohol Abuse						-.412
Withdrwl Iso						.413
Alcoholism						-.587
Neurosis						.227
Diagnosis Deferred						.498

score should not. These factor scores, instead of the individual items, could be used as in input to the AUTOGRP procedure.

If one does not have AUTOGRP available, then the factor scores can be used as a guide to construct mechanisms themselves. For instance, in factor 2, the correlation of sleep, eating, job and mate problems with seizures, convulsions, alcohol abuse and the diagnosis of alcoholism suggests a distinct syndrome present in the population. The institution providing the data, in fact, had a large population of alcoholics and a special program for them. One would expect that any patient with a high score on the alcoholism factor (factor 2) would be on this program, and conversely, any patient with a low score would not.

Another direct statistical technique designed to elucidate which variables relate to a specific dependent variable is multiple regression. In regression, the statistical technique tests all independent variables in stepwise fashion for their power to account for variance in a dependent variable and then, controlling for the intercorrelation effect of the variable which accounts for the most variance, all remaining variables. This procedure is repeated until no remaining variables account for a significant amount of the remaining variance. The technique states in terms of a "multiple correlation coefficient" how much of the total variance has been explained and which items explain it. It is important to note intercorrelations in thie technique, for if two variables are highly intercorrelated, only one of them might appear on the list, for the other would contribute little additional reduction in variance.

Figure 7-9 shows the results of a multiple regression run, where the dependent variable, as before, is whether or not a patient was to be hospitalized. Again, there is striking concurrence in the results obtained with factor analysis, correlation coefficient, and AUTOGRP. The multiple correlation coefficient is .510, which indicates 28 percent of the variance was accounted for by the variables present. This compares with the 33 percent in the AUTOGRP run shown in figure 7-6 using an entirely different statistical technique. Again, the items which appear on the multiple regression may be put in a scale, and mechanisms constructed according to the scores a patient obtains from this scale. By appropriate choice of the dependent variable, which can be any continuous variable or dummied categorical variable, the variables which relate to that particular dependent variable may be studied.

The techniques of factor analysis, multiple regression and correlation analysis are widely available in statistical packages at most computing facilities, often designed for direct use by a social scientist/clinician without the need for professional programming services. Construction of scales and derivation of scale scores are also possible in these packages. Factor analytic programs routinely contain options which print factor scores. The new version of AUTOGRP will eventually contain these options directly at the console, so the AUTOGRPer will have the information available as needed without the necessity of interrupting his work and waiting for output from other sources.

Figure 7-9. Correlations, Factor Analysis, Regression Analysis.   01:46 AM   January 9, 1973

REGRESSION RESULTS FOR DEPENDENT VARIABLE   INPTOTHR   INPATIENT VS OTHERS

STEP 9

VARIABLE DESCRIPTION	NAME	COEFFICIENT	STD ERROR OF COEFFICIENT	STANDARDIZED COEFFICIENT	T-TEST	DF	SIGNIFICANCE	UNIQUE VARIANCE
HALLUCINATE	PROBLEM(19)	-0.1900	0.016	-0.148	-12.24***	6727	UNDER .001	.016
INAPP AFFECT	PROBLEM(32)	-0.2073	0.019	-0.123	-10.73***	6727	UNDER .001	.013
SCHIZO.FUNCT.DISORD	ADX(8)	-0.1883	0.012	-0.169	-15.10***	6727	UNDER .001	.025
SUICID ACTS	PROBLEM(14)	-0.2669	0.021	-0.146	-13.53***	6727	UNDER .001	.020
AGIT HYPERAC	PROBLEM(10)	-0.2404	0.019	-0.143	-13.08***	6727	UNDER .001	.019
AFFECTIVE DISORDERS	ADX(5)	-0.2628	0.018	-0.144	-13.27***	6727	UNDER .001	.019
DISORN MEMRY	PROBLEM(20)	-0.2174	0.018	-0.134	-12.22***	6727	UNDER .001	.016
ANXIETY PHOB	PROBLEM(18)	-0.1399	0.018	0.113	10.45***	6727	UNDER .001	.012
DELUSIONS	PROBLEM(15)	-0.1783	0.019	-0.112	- 9.09***	6727	UNDER .001	.009

REGRESSION CONSTANT   1.921

MULTIPLE CORRELATION SQUARED   = 0.260   F = 262.85 WITH 9 AND 6727 DEGREES OF FREEDOM (P UNDER .001)

MULTIPLE CORRELATION   = 0.510

STANDARD DEVIATION OF RESIDUALS   = 0.333

PARTIAL CORRELATIONS WITH DEPENDENT VARIABLE FOR VARIABLES NOT ENTERED

SLEEP PROBS	PROBLEM(1)	0.020	DEPRES INFER	PROBLEM(26)	0.000
SCHOOL PROBS	PROBLEM(2)	0.093	ASSAULTIVE	PROBLEM(27)	-0.033
EATING PROBS	PROBLEM(3)	0.001	EMOTION LACK	PROBLEM(28)	-0.072
JOB PROBLEMS	PROBLEM(4)	0.061	MATE PROBS	PROBLEM(29)	0.054
ENURESIS	PROBLEM(5)	-0.026	SOMA HYPOCHN	PROBLEM(30)	0.022
HSKPNG PROB	PROBLEM(6)	-0.009	ALCOHOL ABUS	PROBLEM(31)	-0.017
GRANDIOSITY	PROBLEM(7)	-0.068	FAMILY PROBS	PROBLEM(33)	0.059
ANTISOC ATT	PROBLEM(8)	-0.081	WITHDRWL ISO	PROBLEM(34)	0.061
SEIZURE CONV	PROBLEM(9)	0.002			
SUICID THGTS	PROBLEM(10)	-0.015			
SUSPIC PERSC	PROBLEM(11)	-0.029			
SEXUAL PROBS	PROBLEM(12)	0.080			
SPEECH PROBS	PROBLEM(13)	0.041			
OTH PHYS PRB	PROBLEM(17)	0.030			
INAD INTELL	PROBLEM(21)	-0.027			
OBSES COMPUL	PROBLEM(22)	0.034			
ANGER NEGATV	PROBLEM(23)	-0.039			
SPCH DIS	PROBLEM(24)	-0.057			
CHILD PROBS	PROBLEM(25)	0.063			

Besides consideration of techniques available for developing selection mechanisms, there remains the issue of choosing which variable to use. One dependent variable commonly chosen is length of stay. Its importance comes primarily from its close relationship to expense, for cost of treatment is essentially proportional to its duration. It is a striking finding in our study of psychiatric data that length of stay is largely a function of administrative policy and not of disease. This is a reflection of the variability of treatment approaches present in the field. Another useful index is "condition on discharge." Especially for conditions where improvement is expected, it is profitable to review cases where improvement is not the result. The converse is true where improvement is rare. From a mathematical point of view, both these variables are good because they are continuous, although often not normally distributed in the population.

The decision about whether or not to hospitalize is also of great clinical importance. Usually a patient can continue his outside work and family relationships if not hospitalized. Hospitalization markedly disrupts his life and also markedly increases the cost of treatment. Other dependent variables which service as a guide to troubled treatment are discharge against advice, unilateral withdrawal without notice, repeated admissions in short intervals and suicidal or aggressive acts. A large number of internal transfers also often indicates a problem, although there are some preferred treatment paths of multiple units through an institution (e.g., crisis unit to day center to outpatient Rx) which are common and desirable.

Some diagnostic categories usually receive prolonged treatment, and have greater risk of suicide. Acute, first break schizophrenics or older depressives may warrant review on that basis alone. One may wish to check if the symptoms present warrant the diagnosis given. The center itself may identify groups of particular interest. Geriatric patients or patients funded by welfare or Medicare or patients from minority groups may at times require special review. Often, such groups are suggested by a procedure such as factor analysis, which can identify clusters of symptoms, diagnoses and treatment. Cluster analysis, another technique which uses no assumptions of linearity, can suggest populations to review. Experience of a panel reviewing schizophrenia led to the development of a rating scale [6] useful as a means of establishing this diagnosis. Our experience has been limited to non-weighted scales. One would expect greater precision when weighting procedures can be used.

The choice of relevant variables and population to review is not a mechanical or a statistical procedure. It is one which permits broad latitude and challenges the resourcefulness of the clinician and the review committee.

CONCLUSIONS

It has been demonstrated that selecting charts for utilization review increases the efficiency of the process. Mechanisms for selection derived statistically or clinically have equal efficacy. A wide variety of types of mechanisms has been discussed and presented, along with consideration of the data systems needed and the statistical techniques which have proven useful. Lists of mechanisms which have been used have been provided. These were tested only in the aggregate, not individually.

Experience over the course of the project has shown that much more clinical sophistication can be introduced with enhanced information and processing techniques. One spin-off of a review program is the creation of a demand for such a data system.

The future development of systems for selecting charts is likely to be two-pronged. One prong will lead to greater standardization of some mechanisms which will be routinely available via monthly reporting systems to centers desiring them. A second will lead to enhancement of data collected and used for review and the systems to process such data. This will be more urgent in centers which attempt to develop their own mechanisms or in cooperative projects leading to better delineation of standards.

The reason for such emphasis on development of the statistical tools to do the job efficiently is the knowledge that use, utility and interest is much higher if the user is closer to the source. Developing mechanisms to select charts requires the generation of hypothesis after hypothesis, and the process is impaired if the user is not intimate with the details and issues unique to the particular center.

While at this point mechanisms are available for export, it is an important goal to make the AUTOGRP system described available too. A perusal of the list of mechanisms will reveal considerable specificity which hampers generalizability and exportability. While some statements can be made in general, and this catalogue is likely to increase over time, a powerful and effective reporting system close to the user will ultimately provide the best selection of charts.

Appendix 7-A

Selection Mechanisms

A. UNIVERSAL
    1. Recording and retrieval capacity only
       a. reason for discharge against medical advice
       b. all suicides
       c. all deaths
       d. total length of stay greater than one year
       e. admission diagnosis missing
       f. admission diagnosis missing and still in treatment
       g. admission diagnosis missing and length of stay greater than 7
       h. codis = worse and $\frac{\text{disnoref}}{\text{reasondis}}$ = service unavailable or no more
          treatment indicated
       i. adx or codis = no mental illness and totlos greater than 7
       j. adx or codis = no mental illness and termtype = active
          and $\frac{\text{wdmr}}{\text{wdadm}}$ = hospitalization
       k. suicidal (active) and not offered treatment or not hospitalized
       l. ddx = depression or transient situational reaction
          and codis = worse
       m. all patients with greater 4-5 admission in 1-2 year period
       n. ddx = deferred and codis = missing or undertermined
       o. was *not* hospitalized on an inpatient service and has at least one of
          the following symptoms: agitation, disorientation, suicidal act,
          hallucinations, delusions, inappropriate affect, incoherence
       and has admission diagnosis of one of the following: functional
          psychosis, missing, affect disorder, drug dependent, no mental
          disorder
       and duration of illness less than one month

p. presence of delusions and/or hallucinations and/or persecutory thoughts and/or inappropriate affect or disorientation or incoherence and not diagnosed schizophrenic

q. presence of narcotic drug abuse and not adx = drug abuse
presence of alcohol abuse and not adx = alcoholism

r. presence of depression, suicidal thoughts, suicidal acts and not adx = depression
presence of above and not hospitalized if has suicidal act and duration of condition = less than 1 year and/or agitation, or suicact and/or intensity of illness severe

s. those patients whose intensity of illness is severe and not hospitalized

t. adx (schizophrenia or functional psychosis, duration of condition (1 week or less), intensity of illness (moderate to severe), presence of symptoms (delusions and/or hallucinations and/or persecutory thoughts) and not hospitalized

u. absence of alcoholism with adx = alcoholism
absence of narcotic drug abuse with adx = drug abuse

v. presence of sleep, mate, eat and job problems and alcohol abuse and not an adx = alcoholism

w. presence suicidal attempt (act), suicidal thought, depression and not adx = depression

2. Some statistical capability
a. adx = schizophrenic and total los greater than 2 standard deviation from mean
b. all re-admissions for schizophrenia—+2 standard deviation for re-admissions

B. INSTITUTION SPECIFIC
1. Capacity for recording and retrieval only
a. random sample
b. institutions specified forms missing: MSIS admit form, CMHC supple form, ER sheet, PERC, Clin. Transfer form, dictated admit/transfer/discharge summary, change of status form, financial form, progress notes, MSER, physical examination
c. all re-admissions within a given year
d. adx = schizophrenic and total los less than 10 weeks
e. codis = worse and reasondis = unresponsive or no more Rx indicated or disnoref = care unavailable
f. codis = unimproved and disnoref = unresponsive or no more Rx indicated or care available
g. codis = worse and reasondis = withdrew
h. reasondis = unresponsive, totlos = greater than 90 days

2. Some statistical capacity
   a. adx = schizophrenic and totlos greater than 2 standard deviation from mean for a given ward and 2 standard deviation ward length of stay for each ward
   b. codis and 2 standard deviations for adx
   c. codis and 2 standard deviation for adx and ward group
   d. disward = X and totlos greater than 2 standard deviation for that ward

C. RUN SPECIFIC

1. Single mechanism
   a. los by specific ward can be plus 2 standard deviation or interpretation of histogram.
   b. codis = missing and reasondis = no more Rx indicated
   c. adx = depression and codis = worse
   d. adx = trans. sit. dist. and codis = worse
   e. codis = undetermined and reasondis = withdrew
   f. codis = missing and reasondis = withdrew
   g. reasondis = no more indicated and codis = unimproved
   h. adx = schizophrenic and codis = much impr with totlos 30 days
   i. disward = inpt and reasondis = withdrew
   j. disward = inpt and reasondis = service unavailable
   k. adx = schizophrenic and ddx = non-schizophrenic
   l. disward = inpt and number of wards greater or equal to three
   m. termtype = dis and number of wards greater than one, disward = evl, disnoref = unresponsive and age is greater than 21 and reasondis = withdrew or AMA, and totlos = greater than 180 days
   n. general form of mechanism: +2 standard deviation, totlos for term-type and number of wards, disnoref, reasondis, age
   o. termtype = active and totlos less than 10 days, and has delusions or hallucinations or persecutory thoughts or inappropriate affect or incoherence or agitation or disorientation or suicidal acts and adx = schizophrenia/functional psychosis and has not job problem and duration of condition is less than one year
   p. same as above: except duration of condition greater than one year and totlos greater than one year
   q. same as above except: has job problem and totlos is less than 5 days and duration of condition is unspecified
   r. patients within a given admission that have greater than 1 or 2 ward transfers
   s. termtype = discharged and codis = missing
   t. termtype = discharged and ddx = missing, codis = missing

   u. termtype = discharged and totlos = greater than 30 days, codis = missing or undetermined
   v. termtype = discharged, disnoref or reasondis = care unavailable
   w. presence of symptoms and not hospitalized as inpatient: delusions/ hallucinations/perscu/inappaff/incoherent/aggressive disnoref/ suicact/routine impr/duracond less than a month
   absence of all of 10 dx and hospitalized
   tree: presence of absence of 10 dx, diagnosis = psychotic or non-psychotic, duration of condition = greater than 1 week and less than a year or greater than 1 year, codis = improve versus worse, unimproved, undetermined
   x. presence or absence of agit/disorient/suicact/hallucin/delusion/inapp affect/incoherence
   adx = good or bad diagnosis
   duration of condition greater than 1 month, less than one month
   sex
   y. those on alcohol unit with no alcohol adx
   those on drug unit with no drug adx
   z. presence of symptoms not hospitalized as inpatient: agit/disorient/ suicid act/ hallucin/delusion/inapp affect/incoherence
   absence of one of these symptoms and hospitalized, also diagnosis makes differentiation better (i.e., schizo or affect leads to increased hospitalization) age, duracond, intensity of illness and sex (add to whether hospitalized or not)
3. Some statistical capacity
   a. codis = worse or unimproved and totlos = greater than standard deviation

Glossary of Abbreviations

adx	admission diagnosis
ada	against medical advice
codis	condition on discharge
day	day hospital
ddx	discharge diagnosis
disnoref	discharged without referral
disward	ward from which patient was discharged
duracond	duration of condition
evl	evaluation ward
inpt	inpatient ward
inrx	still in treatment
los	length of stay

opt	outpatient service
reasondis	reason for discharge
totlos	total length of stay
wards #	number of wards on which a patient was treated during a single admission
wardlos	length of stay on any ward
wdadm	ward to which patient was admitted
wdmr	ward patient was most recently on

Specification of Mechanisms in a Tree Form

In some instances, several groups are formed from a sequence of variables broken in a specified order. Rather than specify repetitiously the individual values of each group, the order of the breaks is sufficient. An example will clarify this form of presentation

TERMTYPE		WARD OF ADMISSION	CODIS	DIAGNOSIS
a	DISCHARGED	EVL	BETTER	PSYCHOTIC
l		INPT	SAME	NON-PSYCHOTIC
l		DAY	WORSE	
		OPT		
p				PSYCHOTIC
o			BETTER	NON-PSYCHOTIC
p		EVL	WORSE	PSYCHOTIC
u			SAME	NON-PSYCHOTIC
l	ACTIVE			PSYCHOTIC
a			BETTER	NON-PSYCHOTIC
t		INPT	WORSE	
i			SAME	
o				
n		DAY		etc.
		OPT		

CALCULATE TOTLOS + S.D. FOR EACH GROUP

The relevant information in deviation of the mechanism is contained in the order of the variables appearing in the tree, the number of subdivisions formed from any particular variable, and the particular way the subdivisions were formed from the independent variables.

The tree in this example contains 48 branches. In the example provided, all branches are carried out with the same order of variables. More commonly, different variables and different groupings are expected using each branch.

Chapter Eight

Use of Special Studies: The Treatment of Suicidal Behavior

Myrna M. Weissman
Eugene S. Paykel

To this point attention has been focused upon the evaluation of patient care, either from a criterion-oriented perspective or through the analysis of patterns of care based upon aggregate data derived from the clinical record and routinely collected. The present chapter describes the use of special studies as both integral and complementary facets of evaluation. For our purpose, a special study is defined as the investigation of a particular question or set of questions that identify and explicate the character and dimensions of a clinical problem so as to enhance our understanding of the care-giving process and the performance of clinicians in rendering service. Such studies are undertaken to identify gaps and deficiencies both in information related to service delivery and in the actual delivery system itself, to test the efficacy of treatments, to understand clinical decision-making processes and to develop empirical data against which to test normative criteria.

Special studies may be either experimental or observational (nonexperimental).[1] Experimental studies involve the application of classical research design to insure appropriate selection and sampling and to control inputs to comparison groups through randomization. These procedures minimize the existence of chance differences in treatment and control situations and are useful in testing the efficacy of specific treatments or preventive measures suggested by a hypothesis.

This report is based on the work of the Suicide Panel of the Psychiatric Utilization Review Project of Yale University. Eugene S. Paykel, M.D., was chairman of the project between 1969 and 1971. Myrna M. Weissman, Ph.D. was Chairman between 1971 and 1972. Panel members were Carolyn Hallowell, M.S.W.; David Dressler, M.D.; Hal Mark, Ph.D.; Nancy French, M.S.; Donald Shapiro, M.D. Robert Steele, B.D., M.P.H., was a student member; Brigitte A. Prusoff, M.P.H., was statistical consultant; Karen Fox, B.A., research assistant, conducted the interviews and carried out data analysis; Phyllis Newberry, B.A., assisted in data analysis.

Observational studies are more usually applicable to utilization review, as they occur in the natural organizational setting. There is no randomization or control of subjects into treatment, and data collected are descriptive of current practices. In assembling the information to test hypotheses without planned experiments, the investigator identifies natural circumstances that are similar to the problem under study.

The method for selecting the sample and collecting the data in the observational study can be either retrospective or prospective. In the retrospective approach, cases with the specific disorder under study are selected and the investigator "looks back" through the memory of the subject or written documents to obtain information. This method is relatively inexpensive, as time does not need to elapse to make the observations. However, it is a method prone to subjective bias and incompleteness because of its reliance on memory or pre-existing records.

In a prospective study, one starts with the individuals who currently have a specific characteristic and follows the subjects until the outcome occurs. The data, therefore, are less likely to be biased by the knowledge of results, since the data are recorded before the result is known.[2]

This chapter will describe a nonexperimental special study in which record review techniques and a prospective study were used in order to obtain information on the treatment of suicide attempters as part of a utilization review project. Before describing the formulation of the project, a rationale for special studies in utilization review will be presented.

RATIONALE FOR A SPECIAL STUDY

The evaluation of patient care requires a reasonable knowledge about the epidemiology of the disorders under study, namely, the extent of the problem, the population in which it occurs and what one can expect as an outcome given adequate treatment. Judgments about the adequacy of treatment or the outcome should be based on information about the natural history and clinical course of the disorder, the efficacy of the treatments available and the reduction of morbidity or mortality under different treatments. A review of the major psychiatric disorders leaves little doubt that such information is often not available.

Evaluating the treatment of disorders or events that do not fall clearly into one diagnostic group, such as suicide attempts, poses an additional set of problems. For example, information on the prevalence and course of suicide attempts is frequently inaccurate. Efforts to obtain these rates are seriously hampered by the lack of a central registry, as in the case of mortality data, and by concealment. Meaningful comparisons are often difficult to make because of variations between areas or time periods that may be due to the use of different methods for generating data. Many studies focus on only one or two data sources, usually those available, and miss many important potential sources. As a result the literature contains much information about the racial or social class characteristics of suicide attempters which, if used as a basis for planning services, can be quite misleading.

These problems are not solved when one begins to study treatment practices in a particular institution, which is, of course, the main intent of utilization review. A disorder such as suicide attempts may be found in case records under any number of diagnoses or in any number of services. Records are often not systematically set up to record baseline data; follow-up information may not have been obtained; treatment may be inadequately described. These problems are epitomized in studies of suicide attempters. For example, attempters can be found in a variety of services—from psychiatric emergency rooms to medical inpatient units—with any number of diagnoses. The heterogeneity of diagnoses and portals of entry insure that important cases will be overlooked. For example, the more serious attempters may require intensive medical care and never reach psychiatric attention; or the antisocial young adult, for whom suicidal attempt is only one of a number of serious problems, may never be listed as an attempter in case records. In either instance, the magnitude of the problem and the estimate of its care can be seriously misrepresented. Because of these potential sampling biases, quality-of-care evaluation may be based on the typical attempter for whom treatment is standard and relatively non-problematic and may overlook the deviant or extreme case who would require more adequate care.

Where such baseline data are either unknown or not readily accessible, special studies can be an important and necessary first step in developing standards for utilization review. The inadequacy of records in these instances usually requires prospective rather than retrospective approaches. While it is customary to avoid prospective studies, if possible, because of the expense of time, money and staff, in certain instances they are mandatory. With proper sampling techniques and design the cost can be reduced, and such studies can yield a return of baseline information which will be well worth the effort.

This chapter will describe a prospective study that was undertaken as part of a utilization review project to develop criteria for evaluating the care of suicide attempters. This study was undertaken only after the participants had tried alternate approaches. The formulation of the problem and the experience leading to a decision for a special study, the results of the retrospective record review and the design of the prospective study will be described. While this study dealt with suicide attempters, the implications for special studies as an approach to utilization review should be applicable to other evaluation problems in patient care.

THE SUICIDE PANEL

In 1969, one year before the special study was undertaken, an interdisciplinary panel was formed to develop criteria for the evaluation of care to patients with suicidal behavior. Considerable care was taken in the selection of panel members so that a range of disciplines, experiences, expertise and resources was represented.

Included among the disciplines were psychiatrists, social workers, a nurse and a sociologist. Initially, there were seven members; later a public health student with interest in suicide and training in the ministry joined the panel. During the data collection phase a statistical consultant was invited to participate, and a research assistant was hired for interviewing and data processing. Within the disciplines there were persons with research training as well as others with clinical expertise and experience in administration, teaching and/or planning of community mental health services. The different skills did not clearly fall within traditional discipline lines. For example, a social worker and nurse had experience in clinical research; the nurse was also an administrator; the sociologist was expert in mental health service planning.

The geographical locations of the members was another source of heterogeneity. Members were drawn from inpatient and outpatient services, the emergency room, a research unit and a government planning agency. The varied skills, experience, perspectives and locations of the panel members not only led to lively and enriched discussion but were invaluable in providing information on and ease of access to a multitude of resources within the institution. More important, they helped to overcome a tendency towards naivete and parochialism about the total institution and the problem under study.

The panel met regularly, usually two or three times a month, depending on the stage of the project. Minutes of each meeting were kept and circulated before the next meeting. The value of these detailed minutes cannot be overemphasized. They helped to maintain continuity, clarify misunderstandings and keep in focus the task of the members, who were involved on a daily basis in quite diverse activities and might not see one another in the interim. Furthermore, they provided a permanent record of activities and facilitated report writing.

FORMULATION OF THE PROBLEMS

Initial discussions were devoted to defining aims and tasks. These included determining boundaries of the behavior to be studied, where it was to be studied and with what purpose; defining criteria for adequate treatment and outcome against which adequacy of current treatment patterns could be tested; considering the data to be collected from case records and determining the adequacy of records.

Definitions

The most important early task of the panel was arriving at a satisfactory definition of suicidal behaviors. After considerable discussion, review of the literature and some necessary revisions, agreement was reached on the following definitions:

Suicidal Thoughts: Patient admits to thoughts of taking life, in a more than purely speculative or philosophical way, but without gesture or attempt.

Suicidal Gesture: Any act in which initiating moves of a potentially self-destructive nature have been carried out but without the risk of significant physical injury: e.g., climbing onto a bridge or railing, toying with a gun, announcing intent and starting to ingest pills without actually taking more than one or two.

Suicidal Attempt: Any intentionally self-inflicted injury (including by ingestion) unless there is strong evidence both in circumstances and in patient's statements that there was not even any partial ambiguous self-destructive intent. Lack of intent should not be assumed simply on the basis of patient's denial, absence of serious risk to life or added manipulative elements, but would be acceptable, for instance, in attempted abortion by pill ingestion, or compulsive repeated self-mutilation not of a medically serious nature. Accidental self-injury, where unconscious self-destructive intent is suspected, would be excluded because the injury was not intentional.

Scope

It was decided that the study would be limited to patterns of treatment of suicidal behavior in the major portals of entry into the mental health center, as well as field stations and the emergency room. This was not a decision arrived at promptly or without considerable diversity of opinion. Criteria for treatment or outcome proved to be an even more difficult task as it became apparent that sufficient information on the problem itself was not available and that clinical judgments about the degree of suicidal potential were important in the treatment decision and needed to be defined and quantified. As a first step, a series of treatment decisions was delineated such as: treatment versus no treatment; hospitalization versus partial hospitalization/outpatient treatment; treatment modality; length of treatment. Discussions revolved around the components that determine whether each of the decisions had been made appropriately.

Evaluation and Treatment Criteria

Over the next six months the panel began to develop criteria for six evaluation and treatment decisions to answer the following questions.

1. Who should have a suicide evaluation?   An appropriate evaluation regarding suicidal risk should be carried out for patients presenting with any of the following:

1. suicidal thoughts, gestures or attempts;
2. self-inflicted injury such as scratching, slashing, burning or blunt trauma;
3. serious physical injury (not inflicted by someone else) occurring while the patient was alone such as auto accidents, falls, fires and gas;
4. drug intoxication or abuse (including prescribed medications); those who have chronic medical illnesses such as heart, diabetes, epilepsy, arthritis, degenerative neurological disease;
5. drug intoxication or abuse of alcohol, narcotics, habituating drugs;
6. symptoms or signs of depressive illness;
7. overwhelming anxiety of psychotic proportions (sense of impending doom, fear or loss of control) or other psychotic behavior such as schizophrenia, hypomania, psychotic depression, paranoia or acute brain syndromes;
8. severe and acute situational crises such as family discord, loss of environmental or social support, death of significant other, threats to personal freedom;
9. an individual or family history of previous suicide attempts.

2. What should the evaluation consist of?   An adequate assessment of the suicidal or potentially suicidal patient should include attention to the following areas:

1. details of suicidal ideation and behavior—its intensity and history of development, specificity of plan, lethality and availability of planned method;
2. history of prior suicidal behavior;
3. assessment of current symptoms such as depression, hostility, low impulse control, alcoholism;
4. history of recent stresses;
5. relevant medical history, such as history of chronic, serious or incurable disease;
6. social circumstances and resources such as financial, family and friends and their reaction, degree of social isolation;
7. attention to communicative aspects of the suicidal behavior, their goals and whether these goals are being met.

3. Which suicidal patients should be hospitalized?   Hospitalization should be considered for all patients presenting with:

1. a current, clear suicidal attempt;
2. a clear suicidal plan of high lethality, especially if the proposed means are available to the patient;

3. a previous history of suicidal attempts of a medically serious nature;
4. suicidal thoughts or gestures in association with psychosis or delirium;
5. a history of recent marked progression in seriousness of suicidal thoughts or from thoughts to gestures, rather than a chronic longstanding picture without recent change;
6. persistence throughout the interview to express strong suicidal thoughts with intent without being able to see another "way out";
7. an expectation of hospitalization which cannot be changed at interview;
8. an expectation of changes in "significant others" as a result of the suicidal behavior that is neither met nor can be changed appropriately;
9. presence of precipitating factors that cannot be changed;
10. presence of high risk social circumstances such as social isolation.

4. Who ought to be offered outpatient treatment? All patients with suicidal thoughts, gestures, or attempts, where hospitalization is not indicated.

5. Who ought to be offered general medical attention?

1. Any patient where there is a medical problem/lesion other than the most trivial should have appropriate attention or consultation.
2. Hospitalization in medical/surgical units rather than psychiatric ought to be determined solely on the basis of the medical problem and irrespective of psychiatric status: e.g., even if psychiatric hospitalization is not indicated, general hospital might be; if the medical condition would ordinarily warrant medical hospitalization, this should be in a medical rather than psychiatric unit.

6. Who should be compelled to accept treatment?

1. Suicidal risk, i.e., the risk that the patient may harm himself, is recognized widely in legal systems as a justification for compulsory treatment by committal, etc., overriding the person's right to personal liberty. Individual psychiatrists' views do vary, however, as to the degree of seriousness of the suicidal risk which warrants committal.
2. Patients who refuse hospitalization when it is strongly indicated, especially those showing a high degree of suicidal risk, should be hospitalized compulsorily by committal, etc.
3. Reasonable coercion to obtain at least a minimal evaluation should be applied for all patients with suicidal thoughts, gestures, or attempts, even if they wish to refuse any evaluation.

Individual Record Review: Retrospective Studies

With the problem defined and certain criteria for treatment delineated, the panel undertook two retrospective case record reviews. In the first study, 100 randomly selected psychiatric case records were reviewed to determine if the following data were available: criteria variables of suicidal behavior; dependent variables of treatment patterns and potential determinants of appropriate treatment such as sociodemographic variables, clinical status, social and interpersonal relations surrounding the attempt.

Treatment variables were found to be adequately recorded. However, the detailed elements of symptoms, presence or absence of suicidal behavior, previous history and interpersonal circumstances, which enter into the judgment of suicidal intent and might be key determinants of treatment, were either inadequately recorded or were absent.

A review of 500 consecutive recent psychiatric admissions was also undertaken. Any records which indicated that the patients were suicidal by the criteria developed were pulled and reviewed by the panel members as to the adequacy of treatment as defined. A four-month record review yielded only 35 cases showing suicidal behavior. It became apparent subsequently in the prospective study that this was a gross underestimate. Again, many gaps were found in the records. These gaps precluded a definitive resolution of the study in terms of its original aims. A decision was therefore made to recommend the improvement of the records while simultaneously undertaking a prospective study to generate requested data for completing the panel's task.

Recommendations for Record Keeping

In a report by Dr. Eugene Paykel, and the panel members, the following recommendations were made to enable chart review for project needs in the short term and better monitoring of treatment of suicidal patients in the long term.

1. There is at present no way of identifying outpatients who successfully commit suicide while in treatment. The panel recommends that a separate category for closing a case due to a patient's suicide be incorporated into the administrative forms used by medical records, so that such patients can be identified and reviewed.
2. Evidence collected in the emergency room study and from similar studies in other centers suggests that a major dropout occurs between initial emergency room contact and first treatment contact with the mental health center. We therefore recommend that all patients presenting at the emergency room with suicidal attempts or gestures and referred for outpatient or other treatment at the center be identified, and that a clerk check ten days after the emergency room contact to ascertain if the patient came for first appointment and had a subsequent appointment. Those who do not should be reviewed.
3. There is also no way of identifying outpatients who make suicidal attempts while in treatment. Hospitalized patients are identified via

incident reports, and the same procedure should be followed by
therapists for outpatients who attempt suicide.

THE PROSPECTIVE STUDY

The general aims of this study were to document the detailed clinical and social
characteristics, treatment received, and outcome status of a representative sample
of suicidal patients. Specifically, the study had the following aims—

1. To determine the numbers, characteristics, and subsequent treatment of
   suicidal patients presenting at a community mental health center and
   associated emergency services.
2. To investigate the determinants of their treatment.
3. To assess the discrepancy between "good" treatment, as might be recommended
   on the basis of established criteria, and actual treatment received.
4. To determine how the model of utilization review can best be formulated to
   assess the selection and treatment of suicidal patients.

Methods. The general design of the study involved: (1) screening of
the patients presenting at all the portals of entry into the Yale University Medical
Services and identification of suicidal patients; (2) initial evaluation of patients
by a semistructured interview; (3) a one-month follow-up of patients by case
record and/or telephone to determine treatment received and further suicidal
behavior.

Sample and Services. Subjects for the study were patients presenting
within the previous three days with a history of suicidal attempts or gestures, as
previously defined. Subjects with suicidal thoughts without a suicidal attempt or
gesture were not included. The study was limited to patients aged sixteen or
older. Sources of the patients were as follows:

1. The Yale–New Haven Hospital emergency room. This is closely associated in
   its psychiatric services with the mental health center and provided its principal source of suicidal patients. It also comprised the principal acute triage for
   suicidal patients in New Haven and referred patients to other treatment settings. All patients with overt suicidal behavior as defined above were
   included in the study, and not merely those referred to the mental health
   center.
2. Other intake sources included direct admissions to medical and psychiatric
   wards and patients of field stations. Pilot studies of intake sources were first
   carried out to determine the various portals of entry.

Screening. Screening and identification were carried out jointly by the research assistant and the clinicians. Since the main portal of entry for suicide attempts was the Yale–New Haven Hospital emergency roon and most such cases are evaluated by the psychiatric resident, psychiatric residents identified suicidal patients and completed interview forms for those patients. Since one of the panel members was also directly involved in the training of these residents, and another panel member was chief of social services in the emergency room the involvement and interest of the residents was readily obtained. Patients admitted directly to other wards and other services of the mental health center were identified by the research assistant through record screening of new admissions. Every attempt was made to include every eligible subject in the study.

Data Collection. Data collection was as follows:

1. Initial information was obtained by the psychiatric resident immediately on identification when the treatment decision was being made. It covered detailed ratings of mental status and of suicide behavior but was limited to essentials to facilitate adequate cooperation from the busy residents.
2. Further information was obtained by the research assistant at an interview with the patient within the next week, at her office, the patient's home or in hospital, as necessary. This took the form of a semistructured interview covering details of the attempt, circumstances and crises leading to it, previous history, immediate treatment received and patient's perceptions of it. For patients who missed the resident interview or could not be interviewed initially (e.g., patient in coma), the applicable data of that interview were also obtained by the research assistant at this time.
3. One month after the attempt, information was obtained by a follow-up telephone interview and from case records regarding further details of treatment received, patient attendance and further suicidal behavior.

Information Collected: Initial Status (Independent Variables)

1. Administrative variables—name, address, etc.
2. Clinical intake variables—site of intake, day, time, professional orientation of intake clinician, source and mode of referral.
3. Sociodemographic variables—age, sex, marital status, social class, race, ethnic group.
4. Variables relevant to suicidal potential—nature of attempt and medical consequences; availability of means; history of past suicidal behavior; other psychiatric history; current psychiatric symptoms; recent stress; social circumstances including isolation; patient's expectation in regard to hospitalization; reactions and supports provided by significant others; patient's response to interview; Los Angeles Suicide Prevention Center Form assessing suicide potential.

Information Collected: Treatment Variables (Dependent Variables)

1. Clinician's estimate of suicidal risk.
2. Length and adequacy of initial clinical assessment.
3. Clinician's attitude towards patient.
4. Medical/surgical treatment.
5. Hospitalization and site.
6. Recommendations for outpatient treatment; did patient ultimately receive recommended treatment? Where seen?
7. Treatment modalities—ECT, staff.
8. Was treatment compulsory or voluntary?

Information Collected: Outcome Variables (Dependent Variables, Primarily from One-Month Follow-up)

1. Further suicidal attempts.
2. Successful suicide.
3. Social functioning.
4. Symptomatology.

All data were recorded on precoded forms suitable for computer analysis and every precaution was taken to preserve patient confidentiality. Data collection took place between November 1970 and May 1971. However, the incidence of attempts between June and October 1971, was collected so that an annual suicide attempt rate could be calculated.

Cost.   This study required only a modest sum of money, since most of the staff were employed by the institutions and contributed their efforts. One additional research assistant, who worked full time for one year, was hired. She coordinated the study, interviewed subjects, and analyzed the data. The remaining direct costs were for computer time, supplies, publication and a small amount for travel to obtain interviews at patients' homes.

Magnitude of the Problems

Baseline Rates.   Five hundred thirty persons who made suicide attempts or gestures according to the study criteria came to the Yale Psychiatric Services during 1970 and 1971.[3] In 1955, a similar study reported an annual rate of 44 attempts in the same services.[4] The 530 attempts were far in excess of what was expected, and the original plan to interview every attempter had to be altered. Instead, sampling of every fourth successive patient was undertaken so that the one research assistant could handle the interviewing. Suicide attempt figures were obtained from all other hospitals in the area for the same time period, using similar criteria, so that a crude suicide rate for the New Haven metropolitan area could be calculated. This rate was still an underestimation, since private physicians and persons who made attempts and did not seek help were not surveyed. Based on figures obtained from the three major hospitals in the New Haven S.M.S.A., a crude attempt rate of 1.83 per thousand was calculated. (Age and sex adjustments could not be made because the age and sex ratio was not available for the complete sample.) The crude suicide rate for the same period was .073 per thousand indicating that the ratio of attempts to completes was about 25 to one, much higher than the eight to one ratio reported in the literature.[5]

Search for explanations for the increase in attempts between 1955 and 1970 indicated that increases exceeded the growth or changes in the age structure of the population, the utilization of the emergency room or changes in health delivery. A review of studies from Great Britain, Australia and Israel revealed remarkably similar findings as to the increase in attempts over the past decade.

If the 1955 New Haven figures had been used as an estimate of rates, about 45 cases per year could have been expected. If the suicide mortality rates had been used to calculate attempts based on the 8:1 ratio reported in the literature, about 110 cases might have been expected.[a] If the case record search had been used, approximately 105 cases might have been expected. The special study yielded a case rate over five times that of the last two methods. Such a gross underestimate would have yielded quite different and probably inappropriate recommendations for the allocation of treatment resources and staff training. For example, hospitalization might be a possible recommendation for all suicide attempters, as it is in parts of Great Britain, if 100 cases occur annually. If over 500 cases receive treatment annually, there might be considerably different recommendations and allocation of resources. Also one might expect that the 100 attempts noted in the case records might be different in severity and diagnosis from the 400 obviously not recorded. These findings indicated that the magnitude of the problem, based on outmoded information and on the case record search, had been grossly underestimated by the panel. Furthermore, it underlined the value of special study as a mechanism for obtaining baseline data to more reasonably define the extent of the clinical problem being studied.

Characteristics of the Attempters and the Attempts. The majority of attempters were young (69% were under 30); they were single or divorced; females outnumbered males two to one; most were white (73%); they occupied Social Classes 4 and 5 (79%) based on the Hollingshead Two Factor Index of Social Position. The racial distribution was roughly representative of the New

[a]This assumes that the population at risk in the New Haven S.M.S.A. is about 200,000 and the crude suicide rate is about 7/100,000, and is based on the 8:1 ratio of attempts to completes reported by Stengel.

Haven area. The underrepresentation of Social Classes 1 and 2 (8%) probably reflects the use of private doctors by this group. For the majority of patients this was a first attempt. The attempts usually were of mild severity with little intent to kill oneself. They were carried out impulsively, with no specific plan and most commonly by pill ingestion (78%). The characteristics of the attempters and the nature of the method of the attempts were contrasted to studies reported from the United States and elsewhere and found to be comparable. For example, studies from Great Britain, Australia and other parts of the United States showed an increase in attempts over the past decade and noted that most attempters were young females who made mild attempts by pill ingestion.[6] The similarity in findings gave further weight to the reliability of the special study findings.

Methods of Attempts and Special Risk Groups. As described previously, the majority of the attempts were by pill ingestion. Attempters who used pills in comparison with those who used other methods, were younger, were the most impulsive, had the least intent to kill themselves and were motivated towards obtaining attention from significant others. Attempts by cutting and other violent means were more planned, had higher intent to kill and occurred in patients with more self-directed hostility and guilt. While the patients taking overdoses had the *least* intent to kill themselves, they had the *most serious* medical effects.[7]

The discrepancy between actual medical effect and the person's suicidal intent suggests that increasing use of pills has not been accompanied by a corresponding knowledge of their potential dangers. Many of the attempters did not realize the potential lethality of the pills they ingested. This finding suggests that education is needed about the hazards of psychotropic drugs, especially when a number of different ones are taken in combination, and points out the problem of prevention with youthful suicide attempters.

Racial Comparisons. The recent literature describing racial comparisons in suicide attempters leads to the conclusion that differences in nature and severity exist.[8] One problem in these studies is that social class, which may confound results, is not controlled for the analysis. This leads to the erroneous conclusion that attempts are more prevalent and more mild in black patients as compared to white. A review of the literature suggests that most differences can be accounted for by different patterns of care between social classes. For example, the lower social classes tend to use the emergency room for major and minor problems, whereas patients from the upper social classes use private doctors for most problems and save emergency room use for serious crises. The effect of this difference in help-seeking patterns is to see fewer higher class patients in the emergency room but to find that those higher class patients who come to the emergency room have more serious problems. Therefore, the lower attempt rate and more serious attempts reported in the white population may be accounted for by different uses of emergency room facilities. One way to test this out is by studies which control for the confounding variable of social class.

Sixty-two black attempters were matched with 62 white attempters on age, sex, marital status and social class, and were compared on all variables by Steele. Overall, the two groups were remarkably similar on nearly all measures. A few religious and historical differences were found. Black patients were mostly Protestant while the majority of white patients were Catholic. Eighty-seven percent of the black patients experienced death or permanent separation from their father as a child, as contrasted with only 35% of the white patients. Black patients were more socially isolated prior to the attempt. The families of the white patients were seen as more sympathetic following the attempt, while the black families were rated as more indifferent or ambivalent towards the patient.

These data support the notion that racial differences in nature and circumstances of the attempt are inconsequential when social class is accounted for but do not suggest that attention should be given to the delivery of services to the black patients. If external family supports are less available to the black patient, clinicians should be prepared to consider this in the treatment disposition. There may be greater need for hospitalization in the absence of such supports.

Treatment Practices—Gaps in Service

Treatment Received. Most suicide patients (91%), as reported by Paykel et al.,[8] were referred for further treatment beyond the emergency room. However, reflecting the relative mildness of the attempts, only 9 percent were admitted to medical or surgical wards. Of the remainder, the largest proportion (44%) were hospitalized in psychiatric facilities, mainly either a state hospital (45% of inpatients) or the mental health center (34% of inpatients). A substantial group of 38 percent was referred for outpatient treatment.

When determinants and predictors of kind of treatment were examined, considerable rationality appeared in treatment choice. The main determinants for recommendation of either inpatient or outpatient treatment were a set of variables reflecting the patient's severity of attempt. Attitudinal or sociodemographic factors played only a minor role. Follow-up of a subsample of 33 patients referred for outpatient care, however, showed that nearly half did not, in fact, keep their first appointment or get into any kind of treatment. Furthermore, the high dropout rate of suicide attempters referred for outpatient treatment was consistent with reports from other centers. For example, a study of a New York emergency room found that 32 percent of the attempters were recommended for outpatient treatment but only 3 percent actually received it.[9] Independent studies conducted in Melbourne, Australia [10] and in Ashton under Lyne, England [11] reported consistently high rates of poor attendance. Taken together, the findings from New Haven and elsewhere strongly indicate that the follow-up of suicide attempters referred for outpatient treatment requires close attention.

Psychiatrist Countertransference. A 23-item list designed to measure countertransference was included by Dressler et al.[12] This list described the psychiatrist's feelings during the interview with the patient. A factor analysis performed on interviews with 248 suicide attempters indicated that the clinician's feelings towards the patient could be described in three well-defined factors: factor 1—warm and understanding; factor 2—anxious and confused; factor 3—annoyed.

A score was obtained for each patient on the three factors. The factors were found to significantly predict certain aspects of the patient's treatment. Patients were interviewed for significantly longer periods (over 30 minutes) when the clinician felt warm and understanding, and for shorter periods (under 30 minutes) when the clinician felt anxious or annoyed. Patients were more likely to be sent to public inpatient facilities if the clinician felt anxious or annoyed. Medication was less likely to be prescribed over the month following the attempt when the clinician felt most warm and understanding, and most often was prescribed when the clinician felt anxious or annoyed. Voluntary hospitalization occurred most often when the clinician felt warm and understanding and involuntary commitment most often when the clinician felt annoyed or anxious.

The clinician felt most warm and understanding towards the youngest patients, females and patients who made the most impulsive attempts, had the lowest suicidal risk, were the least depressed, made no previous attempts and had the lowest number of previous psychiatric illnesses and depressions. They felt most anxious and confused towards male patients, patients with the highest intent to kill themselves and with the highest potential risk to life, and patients who presented in the early morning.

In summary, clinicians tended to react with confusion and annoyance to the more serious attempters, and their anxiety increased in proportion to the patient's level of psychopathology. They also showed anger towards patients with significant thought disorder and paranoid thinking.[12] These data have implications for utilization review as well as for the training of residents. Since the emergency room resident is the clinician who usually makes the first therapeutic contact with the suicidal patient, training programs need to emphasize the therapeutic role of the emergency room staff. Special attention to the emotional attitudes and personal biases of the staff should be stressed. Since the resident will, according to these figures, see between one and two suicidal patients a day, the problems posed by the suicidal patient should be an important part of the teaching program. The special study identified a clinician response pattern that could work in opposition to idealized treatment norms but could equally be altered through a training or educative rather than programmatic intervention.

Hostility and the Suicide Attempters.   The high "no show" rate for patients referred for outpatient treatment, coupled with evidence in the literature that patients who repeat suicide attempts tend to be patients who do not remain in treatment, is a cause for concern. The attempters were noted in this study and by others to be quite hostile. This hostility was reflected in poor cooperation both at initial evaluation and at follow-up. There is considerable overlap in the social and personal characteristics of persons who make suicide attempts and those who are clinically depressed. Suicide attempters are usually depressed, and depressed patients are often suicidal. Difficulty in regulation and expression of hostility is another characteristic common to both depressives and suicide attempters. Suicide attempters, as contrasted with completers, tend to be young, single or divorced females with problematic and hostile interpersonal relations, characteristics similar to those of overtly hostile depressives who also tended to be young and female. Because of these similarities in age and sex between hostile depressives and suicide attempters, it has been difficult to separate the relative contribution of hostility and depression in suicide attempters. There was need to separate these four variables—age, sex, depressive mood and hostility—in studies of suicide attempters.

Suicide attempters were compared with a group of acutely depressed patients who had not made attempts and were matched on age, sex, social class and marital status.[13] The two groups were comparable on severity of depression, premorbid history and current social adjustment but differed substantially on a variety of assessments relating to hostility. The attempters, as compared to the depressives, were more hostile at psychiatric interview, had more interpersonal friction with a variety of persons including friends, close family and relatives, had more difficulty with the law and more life events in the past year. Other studies comparing suicide attempters and depressives have reported similar findings as to the pervasive nature of hostility in suicide attempters. However, these studies also found age differences (attempters being younger than depressives). In this study we matched on age and still found increased overt hostility in attempters. These findings have preventive and therapeutic implications. The depressed patient with pervasive hostility, especially at interview, is unusual and may be suicidal. The overt hostility of attempters is not related to depression, age or sex, but is related to the characteristics of persons who make suicide attempts. Their hostility makes treatment difficult and may have contributed to their high "no show" rate for outpatient treatment.

These findings have implications for the improvement of treatment. It is important to note that these hostile suicide attempters were as clinically depressed as the patients with whom they were matched, who were receiving antidepressant treatment. The hostility of the attempter may obscure the underlying depression, and the clinician may underestimate its severity and overlook its treatment.

Testing of Normative Criteria

One of the prime aims of the study was to compare the panel's criteria for the care of suicide attempters with actual practice. However, the rich epidemiologic and clinical data obtained from the special study distracted the group somewhat from its original intent which was to test the experts' criteria. Also, some of the findings were unexpected and raised questions about the validity of the initial criteria.

As a first step, the panel focused on a comparison of their criteria for hospitalization with actual clinical practice as found in the special study. This method has been described by Tischler and Riedel.[14] The panel developed nine criteria for hospitalization and translated them into operationalized assessments upon which data had been gathered in the special study (table 8–1). These rating assessments had been incorporated into the prospective study and were completed by the psychiatric resident as part of the interview assessment. Each rating assessment had scale anchor points (usually 4 points) which allowed precise assignment of the patient's behavior.

As can be seen in table 8–1, all of the criteria except numbers 8 and 9, were operationalized. There was some redundancy in the criteria. For example, "a clear, lethal suicide plan" required the same assessment as the criterion, "a current, clear suicide attempt." However, the criteria could be translated into a series of items which then formed the basis of a systematic patient evaluation.

Findings based on these rating assessments were reported by Kirstein, Prusoff, Weissman and Dressler.[15] They showed that the experts' criteria were considerably more stringent than clinical practice. According to the experts each of the suicide attempters had at least one of the criteria necessary for hospitalization and should have been hospitalized. According to the experts, all 248 suicidal patients screened should have been hospitalized; therefore, the 127 cases (51%) who were not hospitalized but had been referred for outpatient treatment would have required utilization review.

In order to determine which combinations of items were most important in actual practice in determining treatment disposition, all of the rating assessments were entered into a stepwise multiple regression analysis. A multiple regression analysis showed that four items: suicidal risk, thought disorder, seriousness of suicidal intent, and medical effect of the attempt were the best predictors of the patient's treatment disposition, accounting for 38 percent of the variance. Patients who were more impaired on these four items were more likely to be hospitalized. Among the four items, the clinical measure of suicidal risk was the most significant single discriminator of outcome.

The application of multivariate analysis to a combination of the experts' criteria and clinical practice, rather than the use of experts' criteria

Table 8-1. The Experts' Criteria for Hospitalization and Their Translation into Rating Assessments

Experts' Criteria	Operationalized Rating Assessments[a]
1. A clear, lethal suicide plan.	1a. How specific was the proposed plan execution of it in the attempt?
	1b. What was the intensity of recent suicidal behavior?
	1c. What were the social circumstances of the attempt?
	1d. Using all available data from the interview, what is your assessment of the intent to kill himself?
	1e. Taking into account all the evidence, what was the potential risk to life of the attempt?
	1f. What were the medical effects of the attempt?
	1g. What is the patient's acknowledged overt intent in making the attempt?
2. A recent history of medically serious attempts.	2a. How many attempts has the patient made in his entire life, including this present episode?
	2b. How many suicide gestures has the patient made in his entire life, including this present episode?
3. The presence of suicidal thoughts, gestures or attempts in association with delusions or psychosis.	3. To what extent does the suicidal behavior show the following motivations? a. bizarre motivation b. depressive delusions c. paranoid delusions d. thought disorder
4. A recent progression in seriousness of thoughts from suicidal thoughts to gestures.	4a. How rapid was the onset and development of the present suicidal preoccupation?
	4b. How much do recent suicidal feelings and preoccupation represent a change from the patient's usual state?
	4c. How long had the patient delayed between deciding to take his life and making the attempt?
5. An expectation of hospitalization that cannot be changed at the interview.	5. What is your assessment of the risk of suicidal behavior by this patient in the near future?
6. The presence of high risk social circumstances, such as social isolation.	6. What are the patient's living arrangements?
7. A current, clear suicide attempt.	7. (Same as 1a–g).
8. Expression of strong suicidal thoughts with intent and without seeing any other way out.	8. None.
9. Expectation not met of change in behavior of significant others due to suicidal behavior nor can change be accomplished appropriately.	9. None.

[a]The scale anchor points are not included here. In general, they were 4–point scales with definite anchor points.

alone, yielded a lower number of patients who should have been hospitalized and were not (misclassified cases). By multivariate analysis only 51 of 248 cases (20.5%) were now misclassified, as compared with 127 cases (51%) using the criteria individually.

This analysis raised several questions about the validity of the criteria. For example, were the patients who had not been hospitalized receiving inadequate treatment or were the criteria of the experts too impractical? The poor follow-through of the outpatients suggested that perhaps all suicide attempters should be hospitalized. On the other hand, the panel had been unaware of the numbers of suicide attempters coming for treatment and the large numbers might have made hospitalization for everyone unfeasible. Furthermore, there is some question of the ethics or the value of forcing hospitalization on so many patients.

There is need for validation of the experts' criteria before these issues can be resolved. Two approaches to the validation would be by comparative study and by follow-up. A comparative study would involve an examination of the misclassified and properly classified cases, in order to understand how these patients differed. This approach might give further insight into the clinician's diagnostic thinking. A long term follow-up of misclassified cases, on the other hand, would yield information on patient outcome to answer questions about the validity of the experts' criteria. If the patients who were not actually hospitalized but should have been according to the panel criteria (the "undertreated" cases), had more repeated suicide attempts, completed suicides or more psychiatric disturbance, etc., then there would be good rationale for the conservative approach of blanket hospitalization suggested by the panel. If, on the other hand, these "undertreated" cases had no different outcome than the hospitalized patients, this would suggest that blanket hospitalization of suicide attempters is unnecessary.

In summary, the combined techniques of experts' criteria, multivariate analysis and follow-up to determine validity offered a promising approach to utilization review.

IMPLICATIONS

There is little doubt that the special study filled a gap in information about suicidal behavior which was necessary before a meaningful evaluation of care in this area could be undertaken. The very richness of data was temporarily a source of delay in one of the original goals of the study: to test out criteria for treatment. The evaluation of the criterion approach never proceeded beyond the recommendations for hospitalization. In part this was due to inevitable time-related factors such as relocation of some staff members and additional new responsibilities for others. More important, the data generated by the study suggested that the panel was not so knowledgeable about the problem as they had thought and that their original criteria might require rethinking.

On a substantive level the study showed that suicide attempt rates were high and had been underestimated in the institution; that attempts were primarily, but not exclusively, a problem of young women and, perhaps, were increased by the ease of availability of drugs; that treatment, in general, proceeded along rational lines with treatment disposition related usually to severity of psychopathology. However, there were also important gaps in service. The recommendation for outpatient care often was not carried out by the patients, and the psychiatric residents were annoyed and anxious about treating the serious attempters. Last, the panel of experts was probably more conservative about treatment recommendations when in an armchair than when involved in the daily decisions, as it was unlikely that any of them really believed that all suicide attempters should be hospitalized.

This study had some immediate impact on the delivery of service and the training of staff in the institution. A log of referrals and active telephone follow-up was instituted in the emergency room so that fewer outpatients would be lost to treatment. There were shifts in the training focus so that more information on suicide attempts has been incorporated into the training program of residents and emergency room staff. There is more awareness of the suicidal behavior of patients coming to the facilities as shown by frequent requests for panel members to talk on the subject to new staff. In this way, these data have been incorporated into the training and treatment programs of the institution. Whether such information results in better patient care can, of course, only be speculated upon. However, without this basic information any effort to evaluate the quality of care of patients with the problem would have been at best, naive and at worst, misleading. Despite the limitations of cost, time and the undeniable distraction of the panel from its original task, our experience fully supports the value of a special study as an initial approach to utilization review in areas of psychiatric care which are uncharted.

Chapter Nine

Outcome Studies

Carol Schwartz
Jerome K. Myers

Outcome assessment is a major component in any comprehensive approach to patient care evaluation.[1-3] This dimension of evaluation relates to the primary goal of treatment, which is to make the patient better. Utilization review procedures described in other chapters of this book emphasize evaluation of the treatment process. While process evaluation is crucial for an investigation of treatment effectiveness, assessment of patient status after treatment has terminated is vital in order to know the end result of patient care.

Outcome assessment fits into an overall plan of patient care evaluation in a number of important ways. At any given point the state of the art in psychiatry—or in any clinical discipline for that matter—may or may not be able to provide definite prescriptions for treatment of specific conditions. When agreement on treatment among experts in the field is low, outcome studies can be used to test or provide a measure of external validity for the normative criteria accruing from expert opinion.[4] Such studies can be conducted at one time or they can be ongoing in connection with a computerized record keeping system. Since the common denominator in all outcome research is examination of patient groups after discharge from treatment, findings can serve the dual purpose of providing useful information to administrators and health care planners while contributing new knowledge to our understanding of the nature of illness and the effectiveness of treatment.[5]

There are some instances when outcome studies can be set up to investigate specific problems of an organization, such as a high rate of dropouts from treatment. Thus, in an area where there may be no available data for evaluating treatment process, outcome assessment can be used to identify gaps and deficiencies in the delivery of care. When an outcome study is designed to serve a trouble-shooting function in an organization, its exploratory nature probably dictates that it be time limited rather than ongoing. It may be necessary to replicate the study at a later point to note any changes in delivery of care resulting from feedback of research findings.

161

Methodological issues in outcome assessment are sufficiently complex to warrant a detailed discussion of research design needed to evaluate the effects of treatment. Outcome evaluation in nonexperimental situations has been the subject of controversy, and some investigators have expressed doubt that outcome assessment can become a routine part of ongoing quality evaluation. Zusman and Ross [2] have argued that a multiplicity of factors besides treatment influence outcome and that random assignment is required to obtain comparable groups of patients. Experimental techniques, such as random assignment to treatment and the use of control groups, are not used in the usual delivery of psychiatric care. A chief characteristic of evaluation research is that it is carried out *in situ*; the subject matter is the pragmatic mixture of treatment that is given in a real life treatment setting.

May, Tuma, and Kraude [6], in discussing issues and problems in outcome research, have noted that it is often difficult to obtain reliable and complete data on a patient's progress through treatment and return to the community when they must be gathered from a variety of sources over an extended period of time. In addition, they have underscored the fact that prospective outcome studies are expensive and time consuming. The setting in which most evaluation research is carried out forces some knowing departures from the ideal in adapting to the realities of routine psychiatric life. With limited time and funding, goals and methods must be tailored to sources of data readily available. Very often this results in retrospective collection of data with reliance on that which is reported routinely in written records or other documents that were not compiled specifically for research purposes.

It is with the expectation that controlled experiments of treatment outcome will be feasible only in rare instances that we share our recent experience in conducting an outcome study on schizophrenia which was part of a larger study to develop criteria for patient care evaluation. One hundred thirty-two schizophrenics treated on six inpatient units and discharged to the community were interviewed two to three years post discharge. The many ways in which patients can show improvement were assessed by measuring multiple levels of functioning, such as mental status, social adjustment and role performance, treatment status and consumer satisfaction. Data pertaining to the inpatient treatment episode were collected retrospectively from hospital records. No special staffing was required to provide varying treatment effects; the treatment studied was that which was routinely given on the six treatment units. The units on which our patients received treatment were quite varied, ranging from a three to five crisis intervention unit of a mental health center to a long term psychoanalytically oriented private hospital. In planning this study we grappled with two crucial issues in outcome assessment: (1) the issue of research design in nonexperimental situations, and (2) the issue of obtaining a comprehensive picture of patient adjustment by tapping multiple dimensions of behavior. It is our belief that these important issues in outcome evaluation hold the key to successful research endeavors in this area.

RESEARCH DESIGN

Methodology of Outcome Studies in
Nonexperimental Situations

The controlled experiment is the ideal methodological approach to the conduct of outcome research. For example, Philip May and his associates [7] studied first-admission schizophrenics with no significant prior treatment who were randomly assigned to five treatment groups, including control. Assessment— consisting of clinical evaluation and use of standardized instruments—was done before assignment to treatment, at intervals during treatment, at discharge and at intervals after discharge.

Outcome evaluation in nonexperimental situations falls short of the ideal in several important ways. For example, the retrospective nature of our study required that we collect data pertaining to the inpatient phase from written hospital records. Limited time and funding forced us to choose a single point at which to assess status at outcome. In addition, we had no control or "no treatment" group, and we lacked random assignment to treatment groups. Indeed our limitations are probably typical of those encountered by researchers attempting evaluation outside of the laboratory or controlled setting. We made every attempt to deal with our shortcomings through approximation of experimental design in data collection and analysis.

Approximating Experimental Design in
Data Collection

When the relationship of treatment to outcome of treatment is explored the following data are required: (1) a clear definition of the study group, which includes establishment of the diagnostic validity of the sample, (2) an assessment of patient status prior to treatment, (3) sociodemographic and symptom characteristics of patients belonging to various treatment groups, (4) descriptive characteristics of treatment and (5) an assessment of patient status at termination of treatment. (See table 9–1.) In a prospective study, data are systematically gathered as the patient progresses through his treatment experience. In a retrospective study, however, the investigator must reach back in time to gather relevant data. In our case this meant that hospital records had to be used to piece together needed bits of information. Consequently, we were forced to rely on types of data that are likely to be reported routinely in written records, such as diagnosis, symptomatology and treatment history. These data were usually drawn from the clinicians' dictated admission and discharge summaries. In using this data source, we made the assumption that clinicians recorded the most relevent aspects of observed behavior in their notes.

Although we found the hospital records somewhat unsatisfactory, the record systems we used were largely handwritten. Since most ongoing psychiatric evaluation research activities, such as utilization review, are heavily dependent upon the written record, this data source is destined for improvement.

Table 9–1. Approximating Experimental Design in Outcome Research

Research Design	Sample Selection	Assessment of Condition Prior to Treatment	Assignment to Treatment	Characteristics of Treatment	Assessment at Termination of Treatment	Assessment at Follow-Up
Experiment	Define Group and Establish Diagnostic Validity of Sample with Clinician Diagnosis and Diagnostic Assessment Instrument	Measure T_1 with Standardized Measures of Mental Status and Social Adjustment	Random Assignment to Treatment	Measure or Describe Treatment Variables: Length of Stay; Type of Unit: Inpatient Outpatient; Treatment Modality, Drug Milieu; Psychotherapy: Individual Group Family; Staff-Patient Ratio; Staffing Patterns; Treatment Ideology	Measure T_2 with Standardized Measures of Mental Status and Social Adjustment	1. Mental Status 2. Social Adjustment and Role Performance 3. Treatment Status 4. Consumer Satisfaction
Prospective Survey		Symptoms as Noted in Record or Computerized Form Assessing Mental Status and Social Adjustment	Document Group Characteristics: 1. Socio-demographic Factors 2. Prognostic Criteria 3. Indicators of Chronicity		Type of Discharge; Condition upon Discharge or Computerized Form Assessing Mental Status and Social Adjustment	
Retrospective Survey						

Systematic monitoring of large numbers of cases can hardly be done without an automated record keeping system. Computerized record keeping systems, with standardized forms for the routine assessment of mental status, role performance, diagnosis and presenting problems, markedly increase the level and amount of systematic data available in records. Increasingly, psychiatric administrators will place high value on their use.

Defining the Study Group. Defining the group to be studied is an important first step in the research process and depends on the specific goals that the research is designed to achieve. In our study we focused on correlates of adjustment in the community in order to fulfill our mandate to develop criteria for patient care evaluation. We studied only those patients who were discharged to the community and who were living in the community at the time of interview. By not studying patients who were transferred directly to another inpatient setting, we eliminated a consideration of schizophrenics who might follow a chronic inpatient course. However, we wanted to know the extent to which schizophrenics use an inpatient setting as a "revolving door"; therefore we made no attempt to exclude multiple admission schizophrenics or those who were rehospitalized.

When the study group is clearly defined, an attempt can be made to establish some homogeneity in the sample or to isolate distinct subgroups which can be examined in data analysis. Criteria for establishing diagnostic validity are totally ignored in too many outcome studies; and despite a plethora of clinical outcome studies of schizophrenia, few have indicated which symptoms or symptom complex were studied. Most outcome reports do not indicate how a diagnosis of schizophrenia was arrived at, other than to note that the patients were diagnosed by a psychiatrist or group of psychiatrists. Needless to say, a lack of pertinent data with regard to specific symptoms weakens the validity of the outcome findings. Owing to the fact that schizophrenia is thought to have a poorer outcome in general than other illnesses with similar symptoms, such as psychotic depression, the results of a study will be seriously biased if non-schizophrenics are not excluded. Similarly, if all schizophrenics are not included in an outcome study, the total picture will be distorted.

The need to achieve diagnostic uniformity is of particular importance if more than one treatment unit or agency is being studied. In light of recent findings relating diagnostic patterns to culture [8], it is possible that varying units or agencies make use of differing criteria in diagnosing illness. This problem was especially apparent to us in selecting our sample of schizophrenics from six different treatment units. We noted that not all patients with a chart diagnosis of schizophrenia necessarily displayed similar symptoms. Through collaboration with a group of Yale psychiatrists and psychologists we developed an instrument for the diagnosis of schizophrenia. The New Haven Schizophrenia Index [9] weights the primary and secondary symptoms of the illness and requires a minimum score, including the presence of at least one cardinal symptom, to adequately establish the diagnosis. Similar research instruments can be developed for other diagnostic categories. Spitzer and Endicott [10] have already experimented with the use of computer generated diagnostic schemes which could be used as a mechanism in sample selection for outcome studies.

Assessment of Condition Prior to Treatment. When the experimental approach is utilized, patients are assessed on important dimensions of behavior before being exposed to treatment. For example, in the Klerman study on depression [11], patients were assessed with standardized measures of mental status and social adjustment before being assigned to treatment groups.

In our study it was not possible to obtain a standardized measure of severity from the records. This would have been possible if all six treatment units had used the same computerized mental status form in routine assessments at admission. We collected information on the presence or absence at admission of such symptoms of schizophrenia as delusions or hallucinations, for the New Haven Schizophrenia Index (NHSI). The symptoms in and of themselves served as a pretreatment measure of schizophrenia. In addition, we devised a total NHSI score which served as a measure of severity.

Assignment to Treatment. Random assignment to treatment groups eliminates systematic biases and permits an objective test of the effects of treatment. When randomization techniques are not used, it becomes important to look at the characteristics of members of natural treatment groups. Such characteristics are then controlled for in data analysis.

In testing the hypothesis that treatment affects outcome, alternative hypotheses relating factors other than treatment to outcome must be explored. Regardless of whether random assignment to treatment was part of the research design, sociodemographic data such as age, social class, race and sex must be looked at, since it is possible that patient characteristics explain outcome more clearly than does treatment.

The natural history of psychiatric illness can strongly influence its outcome. Researchers in schizophrenia, such as Vaillant [12,13] and Stephens and Astrup, [14] have related outcome of the illness to certain of its intrinsic characteristics, such as symptoms of confusion and depression and whether the onset of illness was acute or insidious. To explore this in our study we collected data on Vaillant's seven prognostic criteria [15], the presence of which have been found to be associated with a good outcome. In addition, we gathered data on age at onset of the illness, and number and type of inpatient and outpatient treatment episodes prior to the index episode in order to have a measure of chronicity.

Characteristics of Treatment. Any study of the relationship of treatment to its outcome requires careful documentation of the treatment process. The psychiatric record is a potentially rich source of data for this purpose. Whether data are collected prospectively or retrospectively, one can describe or measure treatment variables such as unit of treatment, length of stay, psychotherapeutic modality (individual, group or family treatment) and drug treatment (type, dosage, duration). If it is known in advance that treatment effects are to be assessed, special forms can be developed for routine use in the psychiatric record. In addition, treatment unit staff members can be interviewed to verify staff-patient ratios and staffing patterns in terms of professional training. It is also possible to study treatment ideology and to contrast, for example, the psychoanalytic approach with behavior therapy in influencing outcome.

Assessment at Termination of Treatment. Prospective design affords the opportunity to reassess patient status at discharge with the same instruments used before assignment to treatment. When this is not possible, written records can be used to obtain categorized data on condition upon discharge ("improved," "no change," "worse") and type of discharges ("mutual consent," "against medical advice," "transferred"), which can substitute as indicators of assessment at termination treatment. With use of computerized forms, it is possible to obtain a routine assessment of mental status at discharge.

The Time Factor in Assessment at Outcome

There is no optimal interval of time from discharge to assessment that can be generalized to all outcome studies. The needs of some studies dictate that multiple assessments be made at intervals after discharge, while the pressures of time and funding frequently allow for only a single assessment. The decision to do a one year outcome or a twenty year outcome depends on the ultimate goals to be achieved. Patient status at outcome can most clearly be ascribed to the effects of treatment when the interval between discharge and assessment is short. The longer the interval the less direct the causal relationship between treatment and outcome. Upon reentry into the community, ex-patients are subject to a variety of stresses and events which cannot be controlled and which can act as intervening variables in influencing status at outcome. It has been found that the greater the number of critical life events or stresses, the greater the psychiatric impairment in a random sample of community residents.[15] Because many psychiatric patients experience multiple treatment episodes, the effects of any one specific treatment are confounded.[6] The advantage of long term outcome studies is that patient careers can be documented and the life history of illness can be explored. Ultimately, it is the long range effects of treatment that are most crucial, and about which least is known. There has been a trend for long term outcome studies to be carried out on a retrospective basis for the obvious reason that prospective outcome studies require so much time. In choosing a time interval for our study, we opted for an intermediate point of approximately two years post discharge, which we felt would allow us to look not only at the effects of treatment but also at the life history of schizophrenia and its implications for community adjustment and treatment patterns after discharge.

DATA ANALYSIS

The experimental logic that influenced the research design of the outcome study should be carried through to data analysis. Tests of the hypothesis that status at outcome is explained by the differential effects of various treatment interventions can be achieved with analysis of variance, taking a score on mental status, social adjustment or role performance or rate of rehospitalization as the dependent variable. Alternative hypotheses, that status at outcome can be attributed to sociodemographic factors or is a result of the natural history of the condition, can be tested in the same way. The conditions under which treatment influences outcome can be explored in detail by controlling for predictive criteria and sociodemographic factors. Multiple regression analysis can be carried out to analyze the effects of many independent variables in a single test and is a useful way of isolating the most important independent variables. Multivariate techniques are available to deal statistically with evaluation of change when pretreatment and post-treatment assessments of patient status are obtained.[16]

Multiple variables can be handled more easily if emphasis is placed on obtaining measurable variables in the collection of data. Continuous variables, such as scores for mental status and social adjustment, length of stay in days, number of treatment episodes after discharge and percentage of time on drug treatment, facilitate the use of multivariate techniques. However, methods are available to handle categorical variables, such as treatment unit and race, so that substance need not be sacrificed in feeding data into multivariate analysis programs.[17]

Two features of the survey nature of our study design were problematic in data analysis and in interpretation of results. We lacked two important features of classic experimental design, the presence of a control or "no treatment" group [18] and random assignment to treatment groups.[19] The treatment was that given in the routine delivery of care on the six units. Consequently, "treatment unit" in and of itself did not represent a distinct type of treatment. Thus we were forced to examine specific treatment variables separately. Although the units varied on dimensions such as length of stay and treatment ideology, there was considerable overlap in types of treatment given on the six units. For example, 96 percent of all patients in the study groups were given phenothiazine treatment during the inpatient stay.

A unique problem in interpretation of findings is posed when a key independent variable is widely distributed. Previous research has shown that phenothiazine treatment has a remarkable effect on the remission of symptoms in schizophrenia.[7] However, the virtual absence of a naturally determined "no phenothiazine" group in our sample prevented us from exploring the effects of this dimension of hospital treatment. It was our good fortune that we were able to look at the effects of phenothiazine treatment after discharge from the hospital, on which dimension our sample was quite varied. We found that the greater the percentage of time on phenothiazine treatment after discharge, the less frequent the acute symptoms of psychosis.[20] Patients who had no follow-up treatment after discharge were a particularly high risk group. The lack of follow-up treatment after discharge was a unit-related phenomenon, capable of being changed by administrative fiat.

The absence of a control or "no treatment" group is not necessarily a handicap when study subjects are exposed to differing types of treatment interventions. Study of treatment effects in the natural setting, where the treatment variables are not manipulated or controlled, demands caution in study design and data analysis. An effort must be made to select natural treatment groups that are known to vary on specific dimensions of treatment, such as ECT therapy or milieu therapy. If they do not, research efforts cannot go beyond description to explore the causal relationship between treatment and outcome. It should be noted that the wide distribution of certain treatments is common in the natural setting, as in the case of phenothiazine treatment of schizophrenia, where clinicians attempt to implement in their practice the methods they see as holding the greatest promise of effectiveness.

The lack of random assignment to treatment is by far the most serious methodological problem. When patient characteristics are not rendered randomly distributed, the effects of treatment interventions must be assessed in light of careful examination of initial group differences on sociodemographic or prognostic factors. The sample in our study varied widely in terms of sociodemographic characteristics related to type of treatment and to outcome. For example, our findings confirmed the relationship between social class and treatment noted previously [21,22] ; upper classes received treatment on expensive private units while lower class patients were treated at the state supported mental health center or state medical hospital. Consequently, social class is related to all of the treatment variables linked to treatment unit, such as length of stay. We also found that the higher the social class, the better the social adjustment at outcome. Due to the interlocking relationship between social class and treatment unit, we were not able to conduct a thorough analysis of treatment effects on social adjustment controlling for social class. If we attempted to look only at lower class patients across treatment units, for example, we ended up comparing the mental health center with the state hospital, as few such patients gained entry into the private treatment units. An assessment of social adjustment prior to treatment would have enabled us to compare pretreatment scores by social class in order to learn whether higher social class patients were also better adjusted prior to treatment. In examining the effects of treatment on social adjustment, pretreatment and post-treatment scores could be compared, using each patient as his own control. Analysis of covariance of social adjustment scores by social class and type of treatment would reveal whether changes in social adjustment scores were associated with social class, treatment or an interaction of the two.

It should be pointed out that one of the important functions of outcome research in nonexperimental situations is hypothesis development. Findings emerge from a study of heterogeneous natural groups which open up new avenues of research. The complex relationships among social class, treatment unit and patient adjustment at outcome were evident in the fact that patients treated on the private units are significantly younger than those treated at state facilities when they underwent their initial treatment episode. A possible explanation for the better outcome in higher social class groups is that psychiatric difficulties are detected and treated earlier, in contrast to lower class groups, in which the pattern of late first treatment comes only after the illness has already become chronic. The role of early detection and treatment of schizophrenia in determining eventual outcome is an area that demands further study.

A chief utility of outcome research in nonexperimental situations is in isolating correlates of good outcome of treatment. Findings on treatment outcome based on a study design that lack random assignment to treatment are not definitive and await further validation through future work. Such a limitation needs no apology; any single study, experimental or nonexperimental, needs systematic replication before confidence in the research findings is well enough established to have an impact on the clinical practice of psychiatry. In our efforts to isolate the correlates of good social adjustment at outcome, we conducted a stepwise linear multiple regression analysis, taking sociodemographic, treatment and predictive factors as independent variables and our global social adjustment score as the dependent variable.[23] Although social factors such as social class and marital status accounted for most of the variance in social adjustment scores, examination of the variables that entered into the regression equation and their zero order correlations revealed that group treatment after discharge was associated with a good outcome while individual treatment was not. Although the zero order correlations failed to reach statistical significance, our findings tend to support those of O'Brien et al.,[24] in whose controlled study of individual versus group treatment of schizophrenia, group treatment was found to be more effective. The concordance of findings in these two studies, one of which employed random assignment to treatment while the other did not, demonstrates that lack of random assignment does not necessarily lead to erroneous conclusions. The issue of concordance of findings from experimental and nonexperimental studies is a fascinating one worthy of study in its own right. While it is our hope that experimental techniques such as random assignment can eventually be incorporated into the evaluative activities of ongoing service settings, nonexperimental studies of treatment outcome should not be ruled out.

MULTIPLE ASSESSMENTS OF
PATIENT ADJUSTMENT

A consideration of how to measure the patient behavior that is expected to be influenced by treatment is equally as important as the issue of research design in outcome evaluation. Over the years a variety of measures, such as suicide rates, rates of rehospitalization and clinical assessments, have been used as dependent variables in outcome studies. While the lack of uniformity in defining the dependent variable has limited the generalizability of findings from outcome studies, the issue of validity in this area is far more pressing. On a theoretical level it has been assumed that mental health and illness cannot be defined as a univariate phenomenon. Therefore, multiple assessments of patient adjustment have become common practice in studies evaluating treatment outcome. Such assessments are "multiple" in that they often include repeated evaluations of the same overall dimension of adjustment with various research instruments often involving different types of rater [25, 26] ; and they are "multiple" in that they cover a wide array of dimensions of adjustment, such as symptomatology and role performance.[27–30] There is a growing body of literature examining the concordance of these multiple assessments of adjustment in order to more clearly specify the nature of treatment outcome [29, 30] and the multidimensionality of mental health and illness.

Psychiatric symptomatology is the most frequently used empirical indicator of mental health or illness. Mental status is a necessary dimension in a clinical evaluation and is the aspect of behavior assessed in epidemiological studies of the prevalence of mental illness in the community [31–34] , yet it is generally agreed that symptomatology alone is not sufficient in order to determine psychiatric impairment.[35–38] Mental health or illness also encompasses a person's capacity to function in a variety of social roles [39] and his ability to exist in society free of the need for institutionalization. More recently, increased emphasis on the consumer in the delivery of health care has produced a new outcome variable, consumer satisfaction. The satisfaction of the patient and his family with what treatment has rendered is a desired result of the treatment process.

The question arises, however, as to the extent to which these multiple indicators of adjustment are related to one another. Does a high impairment score on mental status necessarily mean that a person is also maladjusted in social roles? Shouldn't low levels of impairment in terms of mental status and social adjustment and no need for rehospitalization lead to a high level of consumer satisfaction? One might think that if the various indicators of adjustment tap the same empirical phenomenon; i.e., mental health and illness, they should correlate highly with one another. A low intercorrelation among dimensions of adjustment may simply indicate the multifaceted nature of the phenomenon of health and illness.

In this section we will present data on concordance of multiple assessments of the outcome of schizophrenia to demonstrate that (1) assessments of the same dimension of behavior with three research instruments and (2) assessments of varying dimensions of adjustment, such as mental status and rehospitalization, can lead to differing conclusions about adjustment at outcome. These data will illustrate that a research strategy geared toward obtaining multiple assessments of patient adjustment is the most useful one at the present time. In addition, these data will show that careful attention must be paid to those dimensions of behavior of most interest to the investigator, as some selection of the dimensions to be measured as well as the research instruments used in assessment will be required.

Concordance of Three Measures of Mental Status

Our sample of 132 schizophrenics were assessed with three different measures of mental status, the Gurin Mental Status Index [40], the Psychiatric Evaluation Form [41], and the New Haven Schizophrenia Index.[9] [a] To explore the extent to which the instruments agree on assessment of level of psychiatric symptomatology, the data were analyzed by categories, ranks and correlations. Gurin Mental Status Index scores were classified into low (healthy), medium and high (impaired) categories of level of impairment as defined by Gurin and shown in table 9-2. The other two instruments were similarly classified. When the three instruments are compared by level of impairment categories, it is quite apparent that the Gurin Mental Status Index systematically defines the sample as more impaired than the other instruments. Forty-eight percent of the sample falls into the high (impaired) category with this instrument as compared to 23 percent with the New Haven Schizophrenia Index and 13 percent with the Psychiatric Evaluation Form. The difference in overall assessment by these three instruments is statistically significant ($\chi^2 = 61.47; p = .001$).

Because one may argue that the predetermined categories "low," "medium" and "high" as defined in table 9-2 may not be comparable across instruments, we ranked scores on each instrument from highest to lowest and divided them into highest, middle and lowest thirds. We then compared rankings on one instrument with those on another. While there is a tendency for the

[a]The Gurin Mental Status Index is a 20-item self-report instrument measuring frequency of occurrence of symptoms on a four-point scale; the Psychiatric Evaluation Form is an interviewer rating instrument which records scaled judgments of a subject's functioning during a one week period. The PEF covers dimensions of psychopathology of traditional interest bearing close correspondence to the mental status examination. Judgments of severity take into account intensity and duration of symptomatology and are made on six point scales from "none" to "extreme"; the New Haven Schizophrenia Index is an interviewer assessment instrument noting the presence or absence of commonly seen symptoms of schizophrenia. The NHSI, which contain 21 items on a dichotomous yes/no scale, formalizes a clinical stereotype of what is commonly called schizophrenia for diagnostic purposes.

Table 9-2. Agreement on Overall Assessment of Level of Impairment in 132 Schizophrenics on Follow-up with Psychiatric Evaluation Form (PEF), New Haven Schizophrenia Index (NHSI), and Gurin Mental Status Index (GMSI)

Research Instrument	Low (Healthy)		Medium		High (Impaired)			
	%	N	%	N	%	N	%	N
PEF[1]	45	60	42	55	13	17	100	132
NHSI[2]	31	41	46	61	23	30	100	132
GMSI[3]	9	12	43	57	48	63	100	132

$X^2 = 61.47$ 4df
$p = <.001$

1. [Low = 1, 2; Medium = 3, 4; High = 5, 6] The range of PEF scores in our sample was from 1–6. The mean was 2.81.

2. [Low = 0; Medium = 1, 2; High = 3+] The range of NHSI scores in our sample was from 0–11. The mean score was 2.23.

3. [Low = 77–80; Medium = 67–76; High = 21–66] The range of GMSI scores in our sample was from 31–80. The mean score was 64.44.

ranking of scores on one instrument to correspond with those of another, differences in ranking by instrument were statistically significant.

The less than perfect relationship in overall assessment among the three instruments is further clarified by examining correlation coefficients. The instruments with the most divergent assessments of symptomatology are the Gurin Mental Status Index and the New Haven Schizophrenia Index ($R = .55$). However, the two most similar instruments in overall assessment are the Psychiatric Evaluation Form and the New Haven Schizophrenia Index ($R = .67$).

Data analysis of the three instruments by categories, ranks and correlations clearly revealed a lack of agreement in assessment of overall level of impairment. A factor analysis of the symptom items on the three instruments explained the divergence in overall assessment and showed that the instruments tap varying aspects of behavior. The five distinct factors that emerged from the factor analysis—neurotic factor, schizophrenia factor, motor retardation factor, hallucinations-delusional factor and turbulent factor—were correlated with total scores on each instrument.[42] The Gurin Mental Status Index score correlates .967 with factor scores on the neurotic factor. The GMSI measures this aspect of symptomatology almost exclusively. The Psychiatric Evaluation Form, while tapping a significant amount of the neurotic factor, also correlates highly with the schizophrenia factor. However, it is the New Haven Schizophrenia Index that is most sensitive to the schizophrenia factor and to other aspects of psychotic symptomatology measured by the turbulent factor, the motor retardation factor and the hallucinations-delusional factor. The lack of a higher correlation in overall assessment by these three instruments is explained by their varying sensitivity to aspects of psychiatric symptomatology.

Concordance of Multiple Dimensions of Adjustment

Concordance of multiple dimensions of adjustment was investigated by looking at correlations of mental status with social adjustment and role performance, rehospitalization and consumer satisfaction. As previously noted, mental status was evaluated with three assessment instruments. Although scoring systems have been developed for each of these three instruments, a single total score on mental status was derived in order to facilitate the investigation of concordance of mental status with other dimensions of adjustment. The factor analysis of the three instruments provided the basis for a new scoring system. Individual scores on the five factors were summed giving equal weight to each dimension of behavior. This resulted in a single new score, the "Summary Mental Status Score," which correlated .523 with the Gurin Mental Status Index, .717 with the Psychiatric Evaluation Form, and .880 with the New Haven Schizophrenia Index. All of these correlations are significant beyond the .001 level. It is this score that is analyzed in examining concordance of mental status with social adjustment, rehospitalization, and consumer satisfaction.

Social adjustment and role performance was assessed with a patient self-report interview schedule developed for this study consisting of 152 items concerning performance and subjective feelings and satisfaction in eight role areas: work (18 items), household (15 items), student (13 items), marital (9 items), courtship (10 items), parental (13 items), extended family (20 items) and social and leisure (54 items). It should be noted that not all role areas were applicable to any single individual. A score for each role area was derived by taking the mean of the scaled response items. The mean of all applicable role areas served as a total score for social adjustment and role performance and is the score analyzed in this report.

The number of times a patient was rehospitalized after discharge was chronicled during the follow-up interview using the patient and a member of his family as informants. These data were later cross-checked with hospital records.

An assessment of consumer satisfaction was obtained with the following question asked of family members:

How satisfied were you with the treatment XXX (the patient) received while in the hospital?

1. Very satisfied
2. Generally satisfied
3. Generally unsatisfied
4. Very unsatisfied

Examination of correlation coefficients among these four variables revealed that there is a high level of discordance in multiple assessments of treatment outcome (see table 9–3). Adjustment in the area of mental status is highly and significantly correlated with social adjustment and role performance.

Table 9–3. Concordance among Dimensions of Adjustment: Correlation Coefficients (R)

	Mental Status	*Social Adjustment*	*Rehospitalization*	*Consumer Satisfaction*
Mental Status (Summary Mental Status Factor Score)	1.00	.631[1]	−.074	.023
Social Adjustment and Role Performance (Social Adjustment Mean Score)		1.00	.100	.166
Rehospitalization (Number of Hospitalizations after Discharge)			1.00	.145
Consumer Satisfaction (Family Satisfaction with Hospital Treatment)				1.00

1. $p = .001$

The better the mental status, the better the social adjustment and role performance ($R = .631, p = .001$). In contrast, low and insignificant correlations exist between mental status and rehospitalization ($R = -.074$) and mental status and consumer satisfaction ($R = .023$). The patient's mental status at follow-up bears little relationship to the number of times he was rehospitalized after discharge or to his family's level of satisfaction with hospital treatment. At any given moment it is impossible to define mental health and illness solely in terms of the need for psychiatric treatment or rehospitalization.

The differential impact of various predictor variables (treatment, natural history and sociodemographic) on adjustment at outcome defined in these four ways was also investigated. We discovered that even though the relationship between mental status and social adjustment is substantial and significant, the same set of predictors has a differential impact on mental status than on social adjustment. The greater impact of treatment variables on mental status suggests that symptomatology is a dimension of behavior that is changeable and therefore highly responsive to treatment interventions. In contrast, the importance of sociodemographic variables in explaining social adjustment suggests that this dimension of adjustment is deeply embedded in the social structure and therefore may be more intractable to treatment.[43]

SUMMARY AND DISCUSSION

In this chapter we have dealt with outcome assessment, which we feel should play a major role in patient care evaluation, particularly with regard to the assessment of treatment effectiveness. When studies in this area are planned, two key issues must be considered: (1) study design in nonexperimental situations and (2) multiple assessments of patient adjustment at outcome. Our discussion of research design highlights some of the compromises demanded when research is carried out in the real life psychiatric setting. We have provided data showing a high level of discordance among outcome variables, illustrating the need for multiple assessments of patient adjustment.

If outcome assessment is to be carried out on a large scale, careful attention must be given to the data required for such studies so that they can be collected systematically in connection with a computerized record keeping system. To evaluate treatment outcome one must have data on the independent variables expected to influence patient adjustment, such as treatment, natural history and sociodemographic factors, as well as the dependent variables, be they mental status, social adjustment and role performance or treatment status. Enough diagnostic data must be available to isolate homogeneous study groups. Depending on the specific purpose of the study, assessments of patients' status will be required at intervals during treatment as well as after treatment has terminated.

The pressing need for data on the immediate, mid-range and long term outcomes of psychiatric treatment demands a new commitment from the discipline of psychiatry. A large scale outcome evaluation endeavor may require special staffing to monitor the quality of data input and to interview patients after discharge from treatment. Indeed, an institution may have to reallocate resources to manage an undertaking of this sort. Outcome research in non-experimental situations can be a vital accompaniment to controlled studies of treatment outcome in the endeavor to compile cumulative data on the outcome of psychiatric treatment. Evaluative research in the natural treatment setting has the potential for serving basic and applied research needs. For example, our finding of the importance of phenothiazine treatment in controlling psychotic symptoms in schizophrenia after discharge (J.K. Myers et al., unpublished data) suggests the need for administrators and clinicians to provide this group with adequate follow-up treatment including medication maintenance in delivering the highest quality of care.

Chapter Ten

The Application of the Criteria–Oriented Approach to the Review of Indirect Service Activities in a Community Mental Health Center

Solomon Cytrynbaum

Up to this point, attention has focused on the review and evaluation of the community mental health center's direct patient care activities. While the bulk of staff time is devoted to such activities, center staff are also expected to lend their expertise to non-center agencies, facilities and community groups or organizations in the provision of indirect consultation services.[a] With respect to such consultation services, the role of the center and center staff is not that of direct participant in either a change process or the provision of patient care, but one of resource to an individual, service unit, organization, community group or other service recipient designated as the consultee. Benefit accrues from the enhanced capability of the consultee to accomplish its primary task, irrespective of whether the task concerns change or service goals.

To date, community mental health center-sponsored consultation activities have largely escaped the kind of careful scrutiny to which direct patient care activities have been subjected. In anticipation of a similar trend towards increased professional and administrative accountability with respect to such indirect service activities, for the past year, several colleagues and this writer have been working on the development of a rationale, data base and set of review procedures for the evaluation of community mental health center-sponsored consultation activities.[b] Our work has convinced us that an effective and feasible adaptation of the direct patient care review procedure for the evaluation of consultation activities must involve the following steps: (1) the development of a conceptual rationale or descriptive overview of the consultation process as a

[a]The use of the terms direct and indirect services is similar to that of NIMH [7] and the terms indirect service, community mental health consultation and community organizing will be employed interchangeably.

[b]The early phase of this work was carried on by the Task Force on Indirect Services chaired by Solomon Cytrynbaum and composed of the following members of the Hill–West Haven Division and catchment: Lucy Coleman, Bob Hoffnung, Mike Levine, Karen Pettaway, John Ringwald, Charlene Smith and Kathy Stewart.

179

means of identifying and defining the critical parameters making up the data base, (2) the creation of a data base and information gathering system to record and display essential information in a manner suitable for evaluation and review, (3) the definition of minimal criteria to be used as standards in the review and evaluation of consultation activities, (4) the development of mechanisms for selecting specific consultation projects for more systematic and in-depth review and (5) the establishment of a review process that not only monitors indirect services but insures that feedback is made available to those with responsibilities for program planning and policy development within the institutional-community network.

This chapter reports on the current status of our developmental work in relation to the above. It is intended as a progress report rather than as a de-scription of a final product that is in place and operative. More specifically, we shall begin by briefly summarizing a conceptual overview for analyzing and classifying the consultation process as well as for identifying the data base and instrument requirements for the review of consultation activities. Then we shall explore the feasibility of applying a criteria-oriented approach to assess the qual-ity (defined in terms of the criteria of appropriateness, adequacy and effectiveness) of various community mental health center-sponsored consultation activities. This will set the stage for illustrating how this data base can be translated into a format we believe to be suitable for the application of the criteria. Finally, we will attempt to demonstrate how the criteria can be applied to the review and evaluation of consultation activities. Since most of our effort has been devoted to the preceding phases, it is premature to report on details of the review process, on the decision-making procedures to be used in selecting particular projects for more in-depth review or on the mechanisms by which feedback to administrators and program planners will be carried out. We begin with a brief overview of the consultation process.

OVERVIEW OF THE COMMUNITY MENTAL HEALTH CONSULTATION PROCESS

We have found it useful to examine the community mental health consultation process from a modified open systems theory perspective. Our viewpoint has been influenced by the work of Jaques [4], Menzies [5], Miller and Rice [6], Rice [11], Newton and Levinson [9] and Nelson and Burgess [8]. We have found these versions of open systems theory particularly useful because they offer a vehicle for ordering and understanding the multileveled complexity and the dynamic, shifting nature of the consultation process.

We begin by subdividing the community mental health consultation process as a temporary social system into three major components. The first, corresponding to the input phase in social system terms, we have designated as *inception of consultation*. The second, which is analogous to the throughput phase we have titled *events and dynamics in the consultation process*. And we have labeled the output phase, *termination and review of outcomes*. Each of these phases is in turn subdivided into components. These components and their associated information requirements are discussed sequentially below.

Inception of Consultation

The inception-of-consultation phase is basically concerned with identifying the personal, structural or systems givens and constraints likely to affect the consultation process at various points, either in a facilitative or disruptive manner. Here we have identified six crucial, interdependent levels of interest and their interrelationships. These are: (1) the individual consultant (relevant skills, experiences, ideology, view of consultation process, status and authority in home base organization), (2) the consultant team (dynamics and development over time, division of labor and authority), (3) the consultant's home base organization (social structure, task priorities, authorization for consultation activities), (4) the target or consultee organization (history of previous consultations, social structure, task priorities, culture, authorization for change and potential sources of resistance), (5) the relationship between the consulting team and consultee organization (possibilities for intergroup mirroring) and (6) the larger community context (political and economic realities, interagency collaboration and competition).

Events and Dynamics in the Consultation Process

The second major component, called events and dynamics in the consultation process, is divided into three interdependent subcomponents: task domain, affective domain and interactive and intergroup processes and developments. Here we are concerned with identifying parameters useful in examining how the work was actually carried out (task domain), the sources of emotionality or disruptive feelings, and how such affect was harnessed to facilitate the work or disrupted the pursuit of defined and agreed-upon task or consultation goals (affective domain), and the major changes and developments at the personal, interpersonal, intergroup and social systems level and how they facilitated or disrupted the work of the consultation (interactive and intergroup processes and developments). For purposes of this chapter, the task domain is of major significance.

Any narrative format used to monitor and record the progress of a consultation must pay particular attention to various task behaviors required of the consultant. At a minimum, these would include the initial contact, contract negotiation, gaining entry and establishing credibility, initial data collection, consultant interventions and intervention strategies, the management of conflict, crisis, and of planned and unplanned critical events, disengagement and termination. These parameters represent an idealized sequence of interdependent, overlapping activities which can be said to characterize the more rational aspects of consultant's work at different points in the evolution of the consultation relationship.

Termination and Review of Outcomes

The termination and review of outcomes phase is concerned with the impact and effectiveness of the entire consultation effort. This includes an exploration of the impact not only on the target organization or consultee group, but also on the consulting team, individual consultants and the home-base organization. This phase of the process is composed of three subareas: achievement of objectives; personal and organizational growth; and consultant-consultee satisfaction. In the achievement of objectives subarea we are concerned with identifying the extent to which primary objectives—originally negotiated and established in response to the consultee's presenting problems—as well as secondary benefits, have been realized by service recipients, consultees and other participants in the process. With respect to primary objectives our aim is to examine and assess the extent to which objectives originally contracted for and planned, as well as unanticipated positive or negative outcomes emerged from the consultation process from the point of view of all primary participants, service receivers as well as service providers. The notion of secondary benefits refers to anticipated or unanticipated gains (at a variety of levels) which are the result of participating in the process or are spin offs from participation in various task activities. These do not, in our view, represent benefits or outcomes originally consciously contracted for, although they may reflect some informal aspects of the original negotiations.

The subarea labelled personal and organizational growth involves the documentation of the availability of new personal, organizational, social systems, or political skills and sophistication with respect to the target organization, individual consultees within the organization, or subsystems within the organization. Similar questions could be raised about the consultant, the consultant team, and individuals or subsystems within the home base organization.

And finally, in the area of consultant-consultee satisfaction, it is not only important to determine whether procedures for obtaining these data have been built into the consultation contract, but also to assess the extent to which various participants at different levels within the consultation process were satisfied or dissatisfied with crucial aspects of the consulting relationship as a temporary social system.[c] With this overview as a background, we turn to a consideration of the data base and instrument requirements.

[c]The presentation of this overview has of necessity been sketchy. The interested reader is referred to Cytrynbaum [2] for a more detailed discussion.

PROPOSED DATA BASE AND INSTRUMENT
REQUIREMENTS FOR THE REVIEW OF
CONSULTATION ACTIVITIES

A criteria-oriented approach to the review of indirect services requires a viable data base that captures the consultation enterprise from inception through termination. Any proposed data base therefore must provide minimal but adequate enumerative and descriptive information on the consultation process as a temporary social system. More specifically the data base must contain: (1) a procedure for recording basic identification information on the consultee and consultee organization, (2) a set of categories for noting initial presenting problems as reported by different consultees, as well as anticipated consultant interventions and consultation objectives, (3) a mechanism for recording the frequency of ongoing contacts between consultant and consultee as well as the type of service rendered, and (4) a process for recording the effectiveness and outcomes of the consultation. To meet these requirements, we propose a data base composed of three basic instruments: (1) The Consultation Project Registration Form, (2) The Indirect Service Contact Form, and (3) The Narrative Progress Record. These instruments will be described sequentially below.

The Consultation Project Registration Form

For each consultation activity undertaken by center staff, a procedure for registering the consultee and for recording baseline identification data is required. The consultation project registration form is intended for these purposes. On this form the consultant is to record during or just after the inception of consultation phase, basic identification information on the consultee, the consultee's sponsoring organization, the consultee's presenting problems and the consultant's anticipated intervention strategies and objectives.

The most recent version of the project registration form is presented in appendix 10-A. Section A of this form asks for information which should allow one to identify the consultee by both name and affiliation. It enables one to classify consultees or consultee sponsoring organizations into such categories as law enforcement personnel, facilities and organizations concerned with alcoholism, mental health facilities not affiliated with the center, health and medical care facilities, welfare and antipoverty agencies, facilities and agencies for the aged, schools, daycare centers or other facilities concerned with the education and socialization of youth, community residents/general public and community service groups.

Since consultation requests frequently emanate from different levels within a sponsoring organization and the question of authorization is crucial, this section of the form also includes a set of categories for classifying the consultee in terms of his position, role and responsibilities within the sponsoring organization. We believe that most consultees can be categorized as follows: (1) consultees with direct service responsibilities, (2) consultees with administrative or managerial responsibilities, (3) consultees with programmatic responsibilities, (4) service-team or task-group consultees operating in a larger organizational context, (5) consultees concerned with an organization's structure and functioning, (6) community consultees concerned with various legal, housing, educational, financial or employment problems or those involved in community change efforts. This breakdown is also necessary because the consultee presenting problems and appropriate consultation objectives and intervention strategies categorized in the next section of the form will vary with the level and function of the consultee.

Once sufficient information identifying the consultee has been acquired, it is imperative to catalog the nature of the different presenting problems for which consultees seek assistance. Generally, requests for consultation services arise from: (1) questions regarding an identifiable individual, client or family unit related to the diagnosis, treatment or disposition of the case, (2) the need for the development of staff or didactic inservice training programs for the purpose of increasing professional competence, skill and effectiveness, (3) concerns with organizational, intergroup and interpersonal tensions and conflicts which impede information sharing and compromise task performance, (4) administrative dilemmas concerning aspects of program planning, policy determination, recruiting, training, operating efficiency and the use of personnel, (5) a lack of technical skills, background, resources or information concerning program development, including technical assistance in the preparation of grants or other funding-related activities and (6) the need to develop an organized approach to problem solving concerning the issues affecting the quality of life within a given community. While not exhaustive, this list subsumes most of the general presenting problems for which consultation services are requested.

For data base purposes, these presenting problems must be translated into a series of more specific subcategories corresponding to different consultees. Section B of the project registration form contains such an initial list of categories for consultees with direct service responsibilities. Similar presenting problem categories have been prepared for other levels of consultees, but they have been excluded from this presentation because of limitations on space. Thus, for consultees with administrative or managerial responsibilities, presenting problem categories usually concern the consultee's style of leadership, difficulties with superordinates or subordinates and inadequate administrative skills or knowledge about social systems. Service-unit or task-group consultees frequently report such presenting problems as ambiguity with respect to the unit's task, division of labor and staff responsibilities, conflict or a lack or communication among members of the unit, dissatisfaction with the team's leadership or decision-making procedures, and problems in relation to administrators or other outside groups. Community consultee presenting problems usually involve various legal, educational, financial, housing or employment complaints related to the consequences of poverty, discrimination, political powerlessness or unresponsive state and local human service agencies.

Once the presenting problem has been recorded, it is incumbent upon the consultant to specify, in section C of the form, the type and level of intervention to be undertaken. Typically, such interventions have three general focuses: case-oriented, staff-oriented and social system–oriented.[d] In a case-oriented intervention, assistance is provided to staff of another agency or organization to help them provide better direct services to specific clients for whom they are responsible. Case-oriented consultation implies that center staff do not assume direct responsibility for the care of the client. Thus, case-oriented interventions aim at increasing the level of effectiveness of an individual service deliverer or service unit with responsibility for the diagnosis, treatment or disposition of a case or group of cases. Staff-oriented interventions involve efforts to improve the skills, knowledge and competence of the individual or service unit consultee, particularly through the provision of a variety of staff training and developmental programs with the intent of upgrading the understanding and performance of the consultee or the consultee's staff. Staff development consultation and group work are two more specific examples of this intervention strategy. The former involves work with a consultee group or organization to help them to develop skills relevant to their programs and the latter represents supportive services provided directly to individual consultees, where individual growth and effective interpersonal functioning are facilitated, but recipients are not considered direct service clients.

Social systems interventions aim at assisting the consultee in program planning and development related to the reorganization or redistribution of resources or services and in the resolution of intraorganizational, intergroup and interpersonal problems that compromise task functioning and program effectiveness. Such social systems interventions may be either organizational-and agency-centered or community-centered. The former are usually directed towards the administrators and staff of a human service delivery organization, the latter towards community leaders, organizations and citizens groups interested in originating, planning and implementing programs or organizational change within the community.

Agency-centered social system interventions, for our purposes, include: (1) program consultation involving work with another community organization to assist them in planning and developing programs they sponsor and (2) administrative consultation where service is provided to administrators (e.g., school principals) in consultee groups or organizations with the goal of changing administrative structures and processes by helping the consultee to understand

[d]These general categories represent a minor modification of those defined by NIMH.[7]

and remedy problems such as poor leadership, authority problems, lack of role complementarity or communication blocks.

Community centered social systems intervention might involve such specific strategies as: (1) community organizing in which consultees are community residents, groups or organizations other than governmental and "official" service organizations and the goal is the facilitation of efforts of citizens/consumers to organize themselves to solve common problems or to gain increased access and influence with respect to institutions which affect their lives (e.g., Welfare Moms, Senior Citizen Action Group, Parents for an Elected School Board), (2) expediting/advocacy, which implies active involvement and intervention on the behalf of a community group or participant of a project or program in an attempt to secure or facilitate service from an organization, agency or individual and requires that the consultant directly communicate with the agency or individual in question, (3) interagency collaboration, which involves the consultant in meeting with representatives of other agencies who are also involved with a specific program or service, in a joint effort to plan or resolve questions centering around provision and coordination of services and (4) advocacy research or research projects, where the main purpose is to facilitate the goals of a community group or organization by providing documentation in support of the consultee's position.[e]

Finally, the consultant should specify the objectives and goals of the consultation project. The format for recording these objectives parallels that of the presenting problem section in that the consultant completes only that section which corresponds to the designated consultee. These objectives should be directly related to the presenting problems, and they should represent operational projections which can serve subsequently as benchmarks against which to measure both the appropriateness and effectiveness of the consultant's interventions. Section D of the project registration form contains the precoded consultation objectives categories for a consultee with direct service responsibilities. Drafts of similar categories for consultees with administrative and program responsibilities, as well as for service unit and community consultees have been prepared. We shall return to the question of objectives later when we consider issues related to criteria of appropriateness and effectiveness.

The Indirect Contact Form

The indirect contact form is intended to provide basic enumerative data on the service activity as it unfolds over time.[f] The form is completed by

[e]See the indirect service contact form in Appendix 10-B for a more elaborate listing of types of indirect service intervention categories.

[f]This indirect contact form is a highly modified version of the comparable MSIS indirect contact form (see, Bank,[1]; and Information Sciences Division, Rockland State Hospital.[3]

each service provider for every indirect service contact on a regular basis. It provides information on the identity of the consultant, consultees and project, the date, manner and frequency of contact, the type of intervention and the number of consultants and consultees present. This information can be key-punched directly and stored for subsequent computer retrieval and analysis. A copy of the indirect contact form currently in use in the Hill–West Haven Division is reproduced in appendix 10–B.

The Narrative Progress Record

The consultation process is hardly static. Once the initial contact has been established and the basic identification data recorded on the project registration form, there is still a need to capture some of the more dynamic and process-oriented aspects of the consultation activity as it evolves over time. For a meaningful review process also requires a narrative or descriptive format for selectively recording more complex information about the consultation. Descriptive information on the following should be incorporated into the data base: (1) the consultant's and the consultee's authorization to contract for consultation services, (2) the availability of required experience, skills and resources, (3) the degree of clarity and consistency in the consultant and consultee expectations and their mutual understanding of the contract, (4) the frequency, type and continuity of task-related contact between the consultant and consultee, (5) the consultant's knowledge and understanding of the consultee's relationship to the larger organization, (6) major individual and organizational sources of resistance to change and (7) the outcome and effectiveness of the consultation.

To accomplish this purpose, we have designed the narrative progress record, which is reproduced in appendix 10–C. The content and organization of the questions on this form are directly related to selected parts of the conceptual overview of the consultation process described previously. We are still undecided as to the feasibility of this kind of a data-gathering instrument and about how this information will be recorded. One possibility is that the form will be completed by each consultant and updated on an ongoing basis at appropriate phases in the development of the consultation. An alternative is for the consultant to be interviewed by an experienced peer or member of the review committee using the narrative progress record as a structured guide upon termination of the consultation. It is likely that both procedures will be tested initially.

Before moving on to consider the development of suitable criteria for review, it is important to note that the data pertaining to inception of consultation bear on the criteria of appropriateness; the parameters identified in the events and dynamics in the consultation process phase concern the criteria of adequacy; and termination and review of outcomes has to do with criteria of effectiveness. With this or a similar kind of data base in place, we are prepared to introduce the next steps in the proposed review process.

CRITERIA FOR THE REVIEW OF COMMUNITY
MENTAL HEALTH CENTER–SPONSORED
CONSULTATION ACTIVITIES

Once procedures for generating an adequate data base are in place, it becomes possible to think about how information can be translated into a format that lends itself to a systematic review of the appropriateness, adequacy and effectiveness of the consultation process. As with the use of the criteria-oriented approach in the assessment of direct patient care activities, the standards being established are not absolute but represent benchmarks against which to assess the quality of the intervention. The concrete mechanism for accomplishing this review is a checklist containing minimal operational criteria.

Before proceeding with the review process, the reviewer must assess the completeness of the information in the total record, since judgments about the quality of service are contingent upon the availability of a fairly complete and adequate information base. For a meaningful review of consultation activities to occur, basic information is required on the identification of the consultee, his position and organizational affiliation, his presenting problems, the shared objectives for the consultation, as well as on any major discrepancies in expectations concerning the consultation process or objectives, on consultant intervention strategies and consultant task activities and on the actual outcomes of the consultation effort. The reviewer's initial task is, therefore, to check the entire record. Seriously incomplete information with respect to any of the above categories would be sufficient justification for either forwarding the record for expert review or returning it to the consultant for additional information. If the information in the record is sufficient, the reviewer then considers the appropriateness of the intervention.

Criteria of Appropriateness

Criteria of appropriateness for consultation activities provide guidelines for accepting or rejecting a request to enter into a consultation relationship and for decision-making with respect to the type and focus of the proposed intervention. Thus, two levels of review and criteria are implied. The first involves a specification of some conditions under which either it is inappropriate for the consultant to enter into such a relationship or considerable caution should be exerted in so doing. The second level of criteria delineates some of the parameters which call for particular types of interventions. We are here concerned with the appropriateness of the fit between the presenting problem and the problem-solving or intervention techniques the consultant intends to apply. First we consider several criteria for evaluating the decision to accept a request for consultation services.

In deciding whether or not to accept a request for consultation, at least three major factors and conditions must enter into the decision-making

process. These concern the questions of the consultant and consultee authorization, the availability of adequate staff, time, financial or other resources and the
extent to which the relationship between the consultee or his sponsoring organization and the consultant or his home-base organization is characterized by
explicit, clear expectations and mutual understanding of the working agreement,
task demands and mutual risks.

It is imperative, in agreeing to enter any sustained consulting relationship, that both the consultant and consultee be clearly authorized to do so by
superordinates or others who have authority in their respective sponsoring
organizations or communities. This we believe holds for individual consultees
with service, managerial and programmatic responsibilities as well as for service-
unit, task-group or community consultees. For example, a consultee with service
responsibilities (e.g., a teacher who requests case-oriented consultation in relation
to certain difficult students) may require authorization to justify this activity as
part of legitimized inservice training activity. Or, if the authorization for a consultation to a service unit or community consultee is ambiguous, ambivalent or
in response to pressures of the moment, there is a serious risk of the project
faltering or being prematurely terminated in the face of the difficulties,
resistances or obstacles to change which inevitably arise. Such, we believe, was
the fate of various student and faculty groups which aimed at changing educational institutions in the late sixties. Similarly, if either the consultant's home
base or the consultee's organization is ambivalent about the consultation objectives, or if the personnel or task priorities of either organization changes markedly,
the viability of the consultation effort may be called into serious question unless
clear and firm authorization has been made.

One way in which the issue of authorization can be concretely
operationalized is by examining the extent to which valued organizational resources are made available in support of consultation activities. For example, in
deciding whether or not to accept a request for major, long-term multi-leveled
case consultation, staff-development consultation and organization-centered
social systems consultation to a school or school system, one must assess whether
a sufficient number of consultants or amount of center staff consultation time is
available, whether the center, as the home base sponsoring organization, is
prepared to support such a massive allotment of resources and whether school
administrators are similarly prepared to free-up adequate personnel, staff time
and financial resources if necessary. As will be seen below, it is not difficult to
translate such behavioral indexes into fairly specific operational criteria.

Other related resource issues are more difficult to operationalize but
must still be noted. Thus, the suitability of the consultant's skills, style and level
of experience must be assessed. And if the intervention requires the consultant
(or team of consultants, for that matter) to work across racial, professional,
cultural or other intergroup boundaries, one must be clear about whether the
individual consultant has the required intergroup skills or whether a suitably

skilled heterogeneous group of consultants can be created. Another resource issue concerns the liklihood that the membership of the consultee and consultant group will remain relatively stable. For example, a recent consultation to a major unit of the state department of children and youth services, which included the commissioner as a consultee, was markedly affected by a change in commissioners resulting from the election of a new governor and administration. These, as well as other resource concerns over which the consultant may have some initial control, can play a significant if not determining role in initial decision making concerning the appropriateness of entering into a particular intervention.

Finally, the extent to which the consultee and consultant have clear and agreed-upon views about as many aspects of the work as possible must be considered in the decision making. For example, it is important that the contractual and financial arrangements be as clearly understood and explicit as possible, that obvious hidden agendas be surfaced, that strong negative feelings concerning previous consultants or consultations not be operative and that the projected objectives for the consultation be mutually seen as relating directly to the consultee's presenting problems.

We have translated aspects of the above issues into several operational criteria varying in degrees of specificity. These are presented in a checklist format below in section **I A** of a proposed checklist for the review of consultation services. Given these criteria and the information already existing in the data base, a reviewer should be able to make an initial assessment of the appropriateness of the decision to accept a request for consultation services.

CHECKLIST FOR THE REVIEW OF CONSULTATION SERVICES

I. Review of the Appropriateness of the Consultation
A. Criteria for reviewing the appropriateness of the decision to accept the request for consultation services
1. With respect to the appropriateness of accepting the request for consultation, does the record indicate that:
   a) The consultee was clearly authorized to contract for consultation services by his/her sponsoring organization as indicated by the availability of sufficient staff time, personnel or other resources. ____ Yes ____ No ____ NA

   (NA = not applicable)

   b) The consultant was clearly authorized by his/her home base organization to make available the necessary amount of time or staff resources for this consultation. ____ Yes ____ No ____ NA

c) The consultee did not report strong
negative residual feelings about past
consultants or interventions. _____ Yes _____ No _____ NA

d) The request for consultation services
falls within the range of the con-
sultant's skills and experience. _____ Yes _____ No _____ NA

If NO to any of the above, the record should be forwarded for
further review.

Next, the review process involves the specification of guidelines for
judging the appropriateness of various interventions. A note of caution is in
order, however, because of the range and complexity of community mental
health consultation activities and because modes of intervention may shift over
time. In reviewing the appropriateness of a particular initial intervention strategy,
attention must therefore be simultaneously paid to the nature of the presenting
problem, the proposed focus and level of intervention and the shared objectives
of the consultation. Several selected interrelationships among the focus of consultation, the presenting problems, appropriate intervention strategies and level
of intervention are outlined in table 10-1 below. For review purposes, these
guidelines or criteria governing appropriateness have been translated into a
checklist format in section **I B** of the checklist below.

B. The appropriateness of the intervention strategies
1. Does the record indicate the
presence of the following?
a) An individual or service unit
consultee with a presenting
problem concerning either the
analysis or management of a
case or group of cases received
service in the form of case-
oriented consultation. _____ Yes _____ No _____ NA

b) Consultees with presenting
problems concerning their
administrative functioning
received service in the form of
administrative consultation. _____ Yes _____ No _____ NA

c) Consultees with presenting
problems concerning their
programmatic functioning
received service in the form of
program consultation, staff
development consultation or
program evaluation research. _____ Yes _____ No _____ NA

d) Community resident consultees
with presenting problems relating

Table 10–1. Criteria of Appropriateness as Applied to Specific Consultees, Problems and Interventions

Consultee	Focus	Presenting Problems or Reasons for Seeking Consultation	Appropriate Intervention/Consultation	
			Level	Strategy
Within Organizations Individuals or service unit with direct service responsibility	Analysis of particular case or group of cases	Problems related to the management of a case, student, etc. such as lack of knowledge, skills, resources, objectivity or complexity	Individual or service-unit consultee	Case-oriented consultation
	Own management or case or cases		Individual or service-unit consultee	Case-oriented consultation
Individuals or subgroups with administrative responsibility	Own functioning as manager or service-unit's functioning	Problems of managing internal or external boundaries or in organization's structure, functioning and effectiveness	Individual consultee, subgroup or organization as a whole	Administrative consultation
Individuals or subgroups with programmatic responsibility	Evaluation of existing programs or the identification and implementation of new programs	Problems relating to the evaluation and/or elimination of existing programs, to the identification of unmet service needs, to the design and implementation of new programs and to the obtaining of resources and training of staff	Program planners, administrators and implementors at different levels within and outside organization	Program consultation; Staff development consultation, Program evaluation research
Within Community Individuals or formal and informal community subgroups or neighborhood organizations	Assessment of community needs and sources of resistance, clarification of objectives, resources and time frame; exploration, implementation, and testing of various social action strategies	Problems relating to poverty, discrimination, unemployment, housing and neighborhood deterioration, and unresponsive state and local government, bureaucracies or human service agencies	Leadership of social action group, community residents, leadership of target organizations	Community organizing; Advocacy research Expediting/ Advocacy

to such social problems as poverty,
discrimination, or unemployment
received service in the form of
Community organizing, advocacy
research or expediting/advocacy. ____ Yes ____ No ____ NA

If NO to any of the above, the actual service or services rendered
should be recorded and the record forwarded for expert review.

Criteria of Adequacy

Criteria of adequacy are intended to identify minimal though realistic,
justifiable and feasible standards against which to measure to the consultant's
performance. Two important qualifications must be noted. First, in reviewing
consultation activities, one requires a time perspective and sense of involvement
in a developmental process. This implies that different subsets of parameters may
be appropriate for understanding developments in response to emerging internal
and external pressures at different overlapping and interdependent phases in the
evolving process. And because the consultative process is responsive to a host of
shifting individual, interpersonal, group, intergroup and community or political
realities, different consultant roles and intervention strategies may legitimately
be adopted at different phases in the consultation process.

The development of criteria of adequacy for assessing a consultant's
performance is further complicated by the temptation to define the qualities of
a professional helping relationship, as is most clearly illustrated in the work of
Norman and Forti.[10] To succumb to this temptation would open up a
Pandora's box of value, theoretical and ideological considerations. For it is also
extremely difficult to translate such qualities, which require a high degree of
inference, into concrete operational criteria of adequacy. In what follows, we
have attempted to sidestep as much as possible of the above by defining specific
consultant behavioral or task performance indexes which can serve as a limited
set of initial standards for judging the adequacy of selected aspects of the
consultant's functioning. Although there is some overlap, it appears that separate
criteria of adequacy may have to be developed and applied to consultation
activities involving different levels of consultees. For illustrative purpose, we will
again limit our discussion to consultees with direct service responsibilities.

With these considerations in mind we have delineated two areas of
consultant functioning for criteria development. The first concerns the questions
of whether the record indicates that the consultant and consultee met often and
regularly enough for the work to take place and whether the consultant possessed
sufficient and updated information on the consultee's case and circumstances.

The second area for criteria development is the consultant's task
functioning as presented earlier in the overview of the idealized task domain
developmental sequence evolving from the initial contact and contract negotiation phase through to disengagement and termination. For example, the adequacy

of the consultant's performance in negotiating the contract can be reviewed by focusing on such indexes as the specification of meeting-time boundaries and the length of the consultation. With respect to the later phases of the consultation process, a reviewer should be able to judge from the record whether termination, review and outcome assessment procedures were carried out. Similar behavioral criteria can be anticipated for other aspects of the consultant's task functioning.

In section **II A** of the checklist below, we present a sample of fairly specific criteria of adequate consultant conduct derived from the above.

II. Review of Adequacy of Consultation Activities

  A. Criteria of adequacy for consultation services to consultees with service responsibilities

    1. Does the record indicate the presence of any of the following minimal standards of conduct during the consultation?

      a) Consultant and consultee met sufficiently frequently and for a long enough period of time so that the specified consultation objectives could be realized.   ____ Yes ____ No ____ NA

      b) The consultant provided continuous service to the consultee in that there is no evidence of long periods without contact.   ____ Yes ____ No ____ NA

      c) The consultant demonstrated his knowledge about the case by either clearly communicating his/her understanding to the consultee, or by referring the consultee to relevant literature or training opportunities.   ____ Yes ____ No ____ NA

      d) The consultant insured that meeting-time boundaries and the length of the consultation were clearly understood in the form or an oral or written contract.   ____ Yes ____ No ____ NA

      e) Procedures for termination and post-termination follow-up were carried out.   ____ Yes ____ No ____ NA

      f) Procedures for assessing the impact of the intervention existed and were carried out.   ____ Yes ____ No ____ NA

      If NO to any of the above, note the reason and record should be forwarded for further review.

The above criteria of adequacy were presented with two other purposes in mind: namely, to illustrate the utility of the conceptual overview in pinpointing parameters for the purpose of criteria development and to demonstrate the kind of criteria we are attempting to develop in relation to other types of consultees and consultant intervention strategies. A number of the preceding criteria are obviously applicable to the review of the adequacy of the consultant's conduct in relation to consultees with managerial or program responsibilities, as well as to service-unit and community consultees, but separate sets of additional and operational criteria remain to be developed. Although we are very pessimistic about succeeding, for the reasons stated earlier, we are currently attempting to develop, for consultees with administrative or programmatic responsibilities, operational criteria for reviewing such aspects of the consultant's functioning as: (1) the extent to which the consultant accepted and respected the consultee as a person and professional (2) established a trusting relationship with the consultee (3) supported his personal and professional competencies and (4) engaged in activities designed to increase the consultee's information-based problem-solving abilities.

With respect to a service-unit or task-group consultee, we are exploring the possibility of developing criteria for reviewing the adequacy of three aspects of the consultant's conduct. These concern: (1) the consultant's level of understanding of the consultee subgroup's relationship and function in the larger organizational context in which it operates, (2) the consultant's appreciation of various risks for consultees based on this understanding and (3) the suitability and timing of more structured techniques or facilitative exercises when these are part of an intervention.

And finally, with respect to consultant interventions in relation to community consultees, criteria are needed as guidelines for assessing: (1) the extent to which the consultant succeeded in managing various potentially difficult interracial, professional-nonprofessional or cross-cultural boundaries, (2) how knowledgeable the consultant was about the consultee and about relevant components of the community, (3) the consultant's ability to incorporate diverse strategies, such as various research or social-action activities, into the overall intervention and (4) the consultant's capacity to contribute to a realistic task focus by supporting emergent community consultee leadership and competence and by binding in non-task–related distractions. The next section introduces the criteria of effectiveness.

Criteria of Effectiveness
Criteria of effectiveness provide a basis for assessing the relative degree of success or failure achieved by the consultation. These criteria can be stated in terms of short-term and intermediate goals and are tied to specific interventions, consultees, presenting problems and objectives. Table 10–2 below

Table 10-2. Global Criteria of Effectiveness for Different Consultees

Consultee	Global Criteria of Effectiveness
Individuals or service units involved in direct service	Functioning more competently and independently in providing direct service
Individuals or subgroups with administrative responsibilities	More effective management of internal and external boundaries; increased problem solving, decision making and rational planning ability; greater job satisfaction
Individuals or subgroups with programmatic responsibilities	Greater sensitivity to programmatic needs and skills in planning, implementing and involving community residents in new programs; plans and offers effective staff training programs
Human service team, task group, organization, agency or program	Increased organizational effectiveness as indicated by greater clarity concerning task, division of labor, and authority relationships; increased openness to immediate environmental feedback and greater staff satisfaction and productivity
Community residents, formal and/or informal groups	Increased resources, jobs, human service programs; greater political influence and responsiveness on the part of state and local agencies; increased political and social system sophistication; more viable leadership and a greater sense of personal power.

provides a convenient summary of global criteria of effectiveness for different consultees.

In the case of indirect services, and consistent with the conceptual overview presented earlier, we propose that the criteria of effectiveness can be assessed in relation to three specific subareas: (1) achievement of objectives, (2) personal and organizational growth and (3) consultee and consultant satisfaction. For the purpose of an administrative review, the area of the achievement of objectives is of major interest. Here, we are concerned with assessing the extent to which primary objectives which were originally negotiated and established in response to the consultee's presenting problems were realized and what secondary benefits were also achieved in the process. With respect to primary objectives, therefore, effectiveness is reflected in the extent to which the achievement of originally contracted-for and planned objectives can be directly attributable to the consultation process. The notion of secondary benefits refers to anticipated or unanticipated gains at a variety of levels resulting from the consultation. Such benefits may not necessarily have been envisioned originally but may be related to primary objectives. The checklist format for the above is presented in section **III A** below.

III. Review of the Effectiveness of the Consultation

  A. Achievement of objectives and secondary benefits

1. Were the planned primary objectives
   of the consultation achieved? _____ Yes _____ No _____ NA
   If No, the actual outcomes achieved should be recorded and the
   record should be forwarded for further review.
2. Were there any unanticipated
   positive outcomes? _____ Yes _____ No _____ NA
   If Yes, specify_____

   _____

3. Were there any significant
   secondary benefits for the
   consultee arising from the
   consultation? _____ Yes _____ No _____ NA
   If Yes, specify _____

   _____

The subarea labelled personal and organization growth is of much less interest to administrators because of the more inferential nature of the underlying parameters. Here one requires the documentation of the availability of new personal, service, organizational, social systems, or political skills and sophistication for individual, service unit, organization and community consultees. Global and highly inferential criteria for consultees with service responsibilities are available [10], and we have developed a similar set of criteria for the other types of consultees. However, much more developmental work is required before these can be specified in more behavioral and operational terms. Therefore, we have elected not to present those parts of the checklist containing these global criteria at this time.

And finally, in the area of consultee and consultant satisfaction, it is important to assess the extent to which various participants at different levels within the consultation process were satisfied or dissatisfied with critical aspects of the consulting relationship. That is, it is important to assess the relative degree of satisfaction from the point of view of the consultee and the consultant with respect to the consultant's and consultee's functioning, the consultation process, the strategies, the quality of the relationship between the consultant and consultee, the various outcomes both of a primary nature and a secondary benefit nature and the extent to which there is a recognition, either shared or unilateral, of the development of additional personal and organizational skills and sophistication. Section **III B** of the checklist contains several proposed criteria of effectiveness operationalized in terms of consultant and consultee satisfaction.

III. Review of the effectiveness of the consultation
   B. Consultee and consultant satisfaction with consultation
      1. Does the record indicate a shared

sense of satisfaction with the
consultation on the part of the
consultees and consultant? ____ Yes ____ No ____ NA

2. Does the record show that the
consultee was satisfied with the
consultant's work? ____ Yes ____ No ____ NA

3. Does the record indicate that the
consultee was satisfied with the
process and development of the
consultation? ____ Yes ____ No ____ NA

4. Does the record show that the
consultee was satisfied with the
outcomes of the consultation? ____ Yes ____ No ____ NA

5. Does the record note that the
consultant was satisfied with
his/her performance? ____ Yes ____ No ____ NA

6. Does the record show that the
consultant was satisfied with the
process and development of the
consultation? ____ Yes ____ No ____ NA

7. Does the record show that the
consultant was satisfied with the
outcomes of the consultation? ____ Yes ____ No ____ NA

If NO to any of the above, note any important circumstances and
forward record for expert review.

This concludes our presentation of the conceptual rationale, the proposed data base, instrumentation, criteria and checklist format for the review of
community mental health center consultation activities. A final note on possible
review procedures is in order. If a satisfactory evaluation of the record of an
entire consultation activity is carried out by a reviewer, then the review process
would end at this point and different parts of the data base could become available for future program planning, training or research activities. If, however, the
record is incomplete or aspects of the consultation process are judged to be
seriously inappropriate, inadequate or ineffective, then the record and accom-
panying remarks should be forwarded for a more in-depth and systematic review.
The details and feasibility of this or other mechanisms for the selections of
consultation projects for further review remain to be worked out and tested. For
the moment we are willing to assume that a multileveled review procedure,
similar to that employed in the expert review of direct patient care cases might
work. An alternative would have an expert peer or reviewer evaluate the record,
discuss ambiguous aspects of the record or the consultant's performance with the

consultant and then forward a descriptive report to an authorized review committee for additional review, recommendations and actions.

To recapitulate briefly. In this chapter we reported on the progress of a recent effort on the part of the staff of the Hill–West Haven Division of the Connecticut Mental Health Center to develop an accountability and modified criteria-oriented review process for center-sponsored indirect service or consultation activities. For this purpose, consultation activities were limited to the general categories of case-oriented, staff-oriented and social system–oriented, with either an organizational or community focus. Such a process we believe requires: (1) an underlying rationale for ordering the complexity of the consultation process and for identifying benchmark parameters, (2) a data base and related data gathering instruments, (3) a set of operational criteria to be used as standards for assessing the appropriateness, adequacy and effectiveness of the consultation, (4) a multileveled mechanism for selecting consultation projects for in-depth review and (5) a procedure for providing feedback to administrators with program development or policy-making responsibilities.

In response to these requirements, the consultation process was conceptualized as a temporary social system which develops over time and involves three component phases; namely, inception of consultation, events and dynamics in the consultation process and termination and review of outcomes. Associated with each component phase were several benchmark parameters. A data base designed to capture the most important of these parameters was proposed. The data base included the following instruments: (1) the project registration form, (2) the indirect contact form and (3) the narrative progress record.

The information in the data base was then translated into a proposed checklist format for illustrative purposes. Several criteria, varying in degrees of specificity, were developed for reviewing the appropriateness both of the decision to enter a consultation relationship and of the fit between the consultee presenting problems and proposed intervention strategies, for assessing the adequacy of the consultant's performance and for judging the effectiveness of the consultation for different levels of consultees. Selected sections of a proposed checklist for the review of consultation activities were presented as a first effort to make available a vehicle for the systematic and detailed review of the quality of consultation activities from the point of view of the criteria of appropriateness, adequacy and effectiveness. Procedures for selecting specific consultation projects for in-depth review as well as other aspects of the proposed process are still to be designed and tested for feasibility.

Consultation Project Registration Form

Date_____

A. *Identification of Consultant, Consultee and Sponsoring Organization*
1. Project name or number_____
2. Consultant(s) name(s) or number(s)_____

_____
3. Date of request for consultation service _____
4. Name of person(s) making request for consultation services:

_____
_____
5. Name of consultee(s) if different from person making request:

_____
_____
6. If the consultee(s) is (are) affiliated with an organization, what is the name of the organization? _____
7. What is the consultee's formal title, position and/or function in this organization or facility? _____

_____
8. Indicate which of the following corresponds to the consultee's title, position or function.
_____ a) Individual with service responsibilities (e.g., clinician, teacher, guidance counsellor.)
_____ b) Individual with managerial, executive or administrative responsibilities (e.g., director of center, superintendent of schools, chief of clinical unit, assistant principal.)
_____ c) Individual with programmatic responsibilities (i.e., program planner, program analyst or evaluator.)

_____ d) Service/clinical unit or task group (e.g., clinical team, reading specialist unit.)

_____ e) Formal or informal community groups or organizations (community board, welfare moms, tenants' union.)

_____ f) Other (specify) _____

9. With which of the following human service organizations, agencies or facilities is the consultee affiliated?

_____ a) Law enforcement agencies, personnel, and affiliated groups.

_____ b) Formal or informal groups or organizations concerned with alcoholics or drug abusers.

_____ c) Non-center–affiliated, general health, medical care or mental health facilities.

_____ d) Welfare agencies or anti-poverty facilities, organizations or agencies.

_____ e) Facilities and agencies for the aged and other similar specialized groups.

_____ f) Schools, day care centers or other facilities concerned with the education and socialization of youth.

_____ g) Community residents or service groups.

_____ h) Other (specify) _____

B. *Consultee Presenting Problems*

1. If the consultee's request for consultation services concerns his/her direct service functioning in relation to a case or group of cases, indicate which of the following more specific service related presenting problems apply:

_____ a) Too large a case load.

_____ b) Inadequate resources available.

_____ c) Needs help with specific problem-solving skills or techniques.

_____ d) Insufficient knowledge concerning dynamics or socio-cultural factors in a case.

_____ e) Difficult or complex case.

_____ f) Lack of experience with this kind of a situation.

_____ g) Inadequate supervision or training opportunities.

_____ h) Other (specify) _____

C. *Proposed Initial Consultant Interventions*

1. Which of the following consultation activities are planned for this intervention?

_____ a) Case-oriented consultation.

_____ b) Staff development consultation.

_____ c) Group work.

_____ d) Program consultation.

_____ e) Administrative consultation.

_____ f) Community organizing.
_____ g) Expediting/Advocacy.
_____ h) Interagency collaboration.
_____ i) Advocacy research.
_____ j) Other (specify) _____

D. *Objectives and Goals of Interventions*
  1. If the focus of the proposed intervention is on the consultee's direct service in relation to a case or group of cases, which of the following more specific consultation objectives apply?

_____ a) To help consultee define and arrange for a more manageable case load.

_____ b) To help consultee learn how to obtain more adequate resources.

_____ c) To improve consultee level of problem-solving skills and techniques.

_____ d) To increase consultee's knowledge about the dynamics and importance of certain socio-cultural factors in the case.

_____ e) To help the consultee unravel and understand a difficult or a complex case.

_____ f) To help the consultee arrange for adequate supervision and other relevant training experiences.

_____ g) Other (specify) _____

Appendix 10-B

Indirect Service
Contact Sheet
(Hill–West Haven Division)

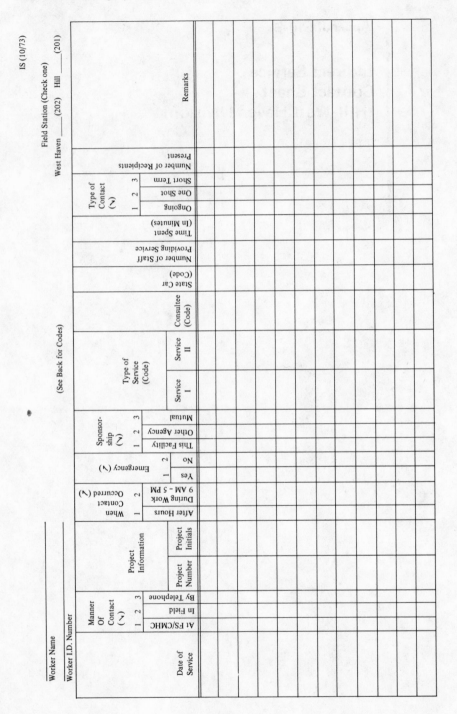

INDIRECT SERVICE

Codes

(a)   *Indirect Service (Codes)*
       —Use two if needed

I.   *Consultation to Other Community Groups or Organizations*
       100   Case-Oriented Consultation
       110   Program Consultation
       111   Administrative Consultation
       112   Staff Development Consultation
       131   Community Organizing
       190   Other Consultation

II.   *Field Station Sponsored Programs and Services*
       191   Ongoing Program Activity
       192   Interagency Collaboration
       194   Preparation, Planning and Review
       195   Group-Work
       196   Individual Work
       193   Expediting/Advocacy/Concrete Service
       120   Public Information and Education

III.   *Services Provided to Own Organization and Staff*
       A.   *Training and Education*
       200   Receiving Training and Education
       250   Providing Training and Education

       B.   *General Administration*
       410   Budgeting and Fund Raising
       430   Personnel Administration
       450   Record Keeping and Routine Data Collection
       460   Meetings for Administration and Organization
       490   Other General Administration

IV.   *Research and Evaluation*
       310   Program Evaluation
       391   Advocacy Research
       392   Process-Oriented Research
       390   Other Research

V.   *Other*
       290   Any Other Indirect Service

(b)   *Consultee Codes*

       Community
       080   Community Residents/General Public
       083   Community Service Group

Professionals
050   Clergy
130   Legal Professionals
140   Mental Health Professionals
170   Nursing Professionals
190   Physicians
200   Law Enforcement Professionals
120   Social Service Professionals

School Related Personnel
240   Principals, Superintendent and Other Administration
250   Teachers
270   Special Service Personnel and Other School Staff
272   PTA and Officers
273   School Board

Students
300   Elementary School Students
310   Junior High School Students
320   Senior High School Students
330   Undergraduates
360   Other Students and Trainees
361   Preschool, Day Care

Governmental
901   City: Mayor, Staff and Officials
905   State: Agency Staff and Officials

Other
900   Other Recipients or Consultees

(c)   *State Car Codes*
1   State Car Used
2   State Car not available, used own car
3   Used own car, did not request State Car
4   Didn't go, State Car not available

Narrative Progress Record

Date_____

I. *I.D. Information*
   1. Consultant name or number _____
   2. Consultation project name or number _____
   3. Name and position of consultee(s)_____
       _____
   4. Agency, organization or group with which consultee(s) is (are) affiliated? _____
       _____

II. *Inception of Consultation*
   1. Has this consultee received consultation services in the past? If so, how did it turn out and were there any disruptive or negative residua?
       _____
       _____
   2. On what or whose authority did the consultee initiate the request for consultation service? _____
   3. If person initiating request for service and designated consultee were not one and same, explain discrepancy. _____
       _____
   4. Was the decision to render consultation services to this consultee in any way problematic for the consultant's home base organization? If so, briefly explain. _____
       _____
       _____
   5. What were the major explicit and implicit reasons for requesting consultation service and what was the degree of clarity about the problems from point of view of the:

209

       a) Consultee _____

       b) Consultant _____

6. Briefly describe any major discrepancies:

   _____
   _____
   _____

7. Briefly describe any important overt and covert expectations of the consultee concerning the consultation process and the consultant.

   _____
   _____
   _____

8. List the consultant's explicit and implicit objectives for the consultation. Any major discrepancies?

   _____
   _____
   _____

9. Describe the consultant's skills, experiences or technical resources which were particularly relevant to addressing the consultee presenting problems and expressed needs.

   _____
   _____
   _____

10. Were there any consultant skills, experiences or resources which were needed but not available? If so, document: _____

    _____
    _____

11. What were the major forces working for change and major sources of resistance at the individual, organizational or community consultee levels assessed by the consultant? _____

    _____
    _____
    _____
    _____

III. *Events and Dynamics in the Consultation Process*

    1. Briefly describe the circumstances and manner in which the following task activities (if applicable) were carried out:

       a) Initial contact _____

   _____
   _____

b) Negotiation of contract _____
_____
_____

c) Establishing consulting relationship _____
_____
_____

d) Entry and establishment of credibility _____
_____
_____

e) Initial data collection and analysis _____
_____
_____

2. Indicate the frequency and briefly describe a typical encounter between the consultant and consultee: _____
_____
_____   _____
_____

3. Discuss the justification for any unusual consultant interventions or for a marked shift in consultation strategies: _____
_____
_____
_____

4. If applicable, how did the consultant manage any major or significant crises, conflicts or unplanned intruding events? _____
_____
_____
_____

5. Document progress or lack of progress towards objectives. How come?
_____
_____
_____
_____

6. What procedures or measures (if any) were employed by the consultant or consultee to assess the effectiveness of the consultation?
_____
_____
_____

7. Were follow-up procedures, consultation alternatives or plans, etc. explored or arranged so that the work would continue after this consultation ended? If so, briefly describe: _____
_____
_____
_____

IV. *Termination and Review of Outcomes*

1. List the explicit objectives which were achieved and not achieved both of a short-term and long-term nature: _____
_____
_____
_____

2. Describe any unanticipated objectives or secondary benefits which were achieved: _____
_____
_____
_____

3. Briefly record any additional evidence bearing on the impact of the consultation on the consultee's level of functioning and effectiveness and why: _____
_____
_____
_____

4. Indicate the extent to which the consultee and consultant were satisfied or dissatisfied with consultant's functioning, the consultation process and outcomes:_____
_____
_____
_____

5. If applicable, what next step or follow-up procedures were agreed upon? _____
_____
_____
_____

Chapter Eleven

Utilization Review Within an Institutional Context

Phillip B. Goldblatt
Jerzy E. Henisz
Gary L. Tischler

Up to this point, attention has focused upon a host of technical and mechanical issues related to both patient care evaluation and psychiatric utilization review. Utilization review, however, is more than a technique or method. It represents a process in which a group of practitioners both evaluate and provide feedback to the institution about the performance of their peers. While the criteria-oriented approach, case selection mechanisms and study techniques advocated in previous chapters may facilitate utilization review, there are also a number of organizational and group phenomena likely to intrude upon and influence this process. These are the issues with which the present chapter is concerned.

As part of the PURE Project, utilization review committees were established in four representative community mental health centers. Observation of these committees brought into focus the commonality of problems encountered and the variety of solutions attempted. In the pages to follow, we shall describe in some detail the issues that surfaced and the institutional processes involved in the growth and development of utilization review committees at those centers.

THE PARTICIPANTS AND
GENERAL METHODOLOGY

The participating centers were quite different in terms of location (urban versus suburban), centralization of services, programs offered, staffing patterns, size, years of operation and funding sources.

Center A opened in 1966 as a joint endeavor of a majority university and the state government. The state is the primary financial support. All top level staff have joint university appointments. The center is located in an urban area serving a population of 400,000 divided into two *catchment* areas. It provides comprehensive mental health services, including three inpatient units; intake and emergency service; outpatient services for brief treatment, continuing care, medication support and rehabilitation; a drug abuse unit; two field stations; a community consultation service; and a training component. Despite this diversity of service, there appears to be a high degree of administrative centralization. The majority of personnel either have offices or receive mail at the main building, although their work may take place in field clinics or in locations outside of the building. At the time of the study, the center employed 230 clinical personnel, of whom nearly 30 percent were medical residents, psychology and social work trainees and other students. The center's total records numbered over 15,000 with an average of 2500 active cases and 4000 admissions per year.

Center B opened in January 1971 under the jurisdiction of the state government. Top level personnel were also on the faculty of a large university and under the auspices of a large university affiliated hospital nearby. This relationship is somewhat less strong than at Center A. Center B is located in an urban area, serving a catchment population of 172,000. It is directly responsible to a local council, made up of all mental health facilities in the area, of which the center's director is also chairman. The center provides comprehensive mental health services, including two inpatient units; services for children and a day school; outpatient services for brief and extended treatment, continuing care, and medication support, and rehabilitation. There are two field clinics which existed some years prior to the opening of the center itself. Although the center operates under a "dispersed and decentralized model," all services except for these field clinics are relatively centralized. At the time of the study, the center employed 110 clinical staff members, a significant portion of whom were also medical residents, psychology trainees and social work students. Its total records numbered approximately 3000, with an average of 1000 active cases and 1600 admissions per year.

Center C opened in 1969 under the jurisdiction of the District of Columbia. It is dependent upon congressional appropriations. Originally, a number of professional staff held joint appointments with a nearby university; however, this is not true at the present time and there is little direct university affiliation. The center is located in a densely populated residential section of Washington, serving a catchment of 240,000 people. Center C provides comprehensive mental health services including inpatient and emergency services at a general hospital which, in contrast to the other centers, is located several miles distant from the main clinic building. The center also provides outpatient services for brief treatment, day care, youth services, and an alcoholism treatment program, as well as community consultation. A number of these services are provided at field locations, by contract agencies, or in special direct affiliation with the hospital. Some services were in operation for many years prior to the opening of Center C. Spread over a rather large geographic area, these services are relatively decentralized. During the course of the study, a number of reorganizations were attempted. When the study began, the center employed approximately 200 clinical staff but suffered greatly from budgetary cutbacks and a job freeze. In addition, there was a lack of clerical and other support personnel. There was an average of 2000 active cases and nearly 3000 admissions per year.

Center D opened in 1969, funded by the state government but under the jurisdiction of a local community mental health board, of which the center's director is also chairman. The center and its professional staff hold no university affiliations. The center is located in a suburban area some distance from any major city and is part of a large complex of health services for the county. It serves a catchment population of 230,000 covering a five-town area. Comprehensive mental health services are provided by the center, including an inpatient unit located in the general hospital of the health complex; intake and emergency services; a variety of services for children; outpatient services for extended and brief treatment; day treatment; an alcoholism and drug abuse program; a rehabilitation service; and two field clinics, as well as community consultation. A number of these services are provided by contract with outside agencies which existed prior to the opening of the mental health center building. There are a great number of units and a variety of services and a high degree of decentralization. The center employed 230 clinical personnel many of whom worked part time. There were no residents and few trainees. Its total records numbered 8600 with an average of 1600 active cases and 4000 admissions per year.

As the descriptions indicate, the participating centers varied a good deal in terms of administrative structure, program, client population, staffing and affiliations. Table 11-1 summarizes the major differences. We were, therefore, confronted by varying organizational contexts within which to explore the evolution of a single process. The exploration itself was largely a naturalistic and descriptive one that made use of data from the participating centers based upon narrative information, questionnaires and interview material.

Each center agreed to keep detailed minutes of all utilization review meetings, including those of subcommittees, following a specified outline (Table 11-2). Further, each agreed to make available all correspondence to and from the committee and to report on regular and informal contacts between the utilization review chariman and his research assistant at the center and any other members of the staff or administration. Questionnaires were distributed to all staff at each center just prior to the committee's beginning its work and one year later to test attitudes toward supervision and review. These question-

Table 11-1.   Summary Table Comparing Centers.

Center	University Affiliation*	Degree of Centralization**	Primary Funding Source	Years in Operation	Catchment Population
A	++	++	State/Federal Matching	7	400,000
B	+	+-	State	2	172,000
C	+-	-	D. of C.	4	240,000
D	-	-	State	4	230,000

Center	Number of Clinical Staff	Number of Active Cases	Total Number of Records	Admissions per Year	
A	230	~2,500	15,000	4,000	(1/3 readmit)
B	110	~1,000	3,000	1,600	(400 readmit)
C	200	~2,000	?N.A.	2,750	
D	230	~1,600	8,600	4,000	

*++ = much direct affiliation, faculty appointments

 + = indirect affiliation, faculty appointments

+- = no affiliation except some faculty appointments

 - = no affiliation

**++ = high degree of centralization

+- = centralization in some areas, not center-wide

 - = loose centralization

Table 11-2. Minutes of Utilization Review Committee Meeting

Name of Mental Health Center _____

Date _____

Duration of Meeting_____ Hours

Committee Members Present	Position at Center
_____	_____
_____	_____
_____	_____
_____	_____
_____	_____
_____	_____
_____	_____
_____	_____
_____	_____

Committee Members Absent	Position at Center
_____	_____
_____	_____
_____	_____
_____	_____
_____	_____

Guests and Observers Present	Position at Center or Additional Info.
_____	_____
_____	_____
_____	_____
_____	_____
_____	_____

1. Have there been developments with any previously incompleted Utilization Review Committee business? yes ( ) no ( )
   If yes
   A. What is the nature of that business? (If an outline of the specific business was included in a previous set of minutes reference only need be made here)

_____

_____

_____

(continued)

B. What has developed? _____

_____

_____

_____

_____

C. Did the committee decide further action is necessary?   yes ( )   no ( )
   Comment. _____

_____

_____

_____

2. Have any incoming communications, formal or informal, been received by the committee since the last meeting?   yes ( )   no ( )
   If yes
   A. What is the nature of these communications? (You may summarize or send copies of written materials if preferred) _____

_____

_____

_____

_____

   B. Did the committee decide action is indicated?   yes ( )   no ( )
      What action? _____

_____

_____

_____

_____

3. Have any outgoing communications, formal or informal, been drafted by the Utilization Review Committee since the last meeting?   yes ( )   no ( )
   If yes
   A. What is the nature of these communications? _____

_____

_____

_____

_____

_____

   B. If action was requested or required, or if recommendations were solicited or contained in the outgoing communications, does the committee feel appropriate response was obtained from the receiving party(ies)?   yes ( )   no ( )   NA ( )
      Please elaborate _____

_____

_____

_____

_____

C. Is additional Utilization Review Committee action indicated?   yes ( )   no ( )
   Comment._____

_____

_____

_____

_____

4. Were any analyses from MSIS, PURE or other sources, included as part of the utilization
   review process?   yes ( )   no ( )
   If yes
   A. Name of report(s) _____

   _____

   B. Were they useful?   yes ( )   no ( )
   C. Were they necessary for adequate review?   yes ( )   no ( )
   Comment as to why._____

_____

_____

_____

_____

5. Is the Utilization Review Committee divided into functional subcommittees?   yes ( )
                                                                                  no ( )

   If yes
   A. What are the names of these subcommittees?
      Sub #1 _____
      Sub #2 _____ _____
      Sub #3 _____

   B. What are the tasks of these subcommittees? (follow numbering sequence)
      Sub #1 _____

_____

_____

      Sub#2 _____

_____

_____

      Sub #3 _____

_____

_____

_____

(continued)

C. Who are the members of these subcommittees, are they members of the Center Utilization Review Committee, and how much time did they spend in subcommittee work since the last UR Committee meeting?

Name	*Position*	*Sub assigned to*	*Hours spent*

D. Summarize subcommittee developments occurring since the last regular Utilization Review Committee meeting.

Sub #1 _____

_____

_____

_____

Sub #2 _____

_____

_____

Sub #3 _____

_____

_____

_____

6. Did individual Utilization Review Committee members spend time other than that already indicated in performing some formal aspect of utilization review?   yes ( ) no ( )
If yes
Please include pertinent information here as to hours, type and purpose of inquiry, etc.

_____

_____

_____

_____

_____

_____

7. Please comment on major arenas of discussion presented at this meeting in which the Utilization Review Committee members can be said to have:
A. Attained agreement. _____

_____

_____

_____

_____

B. Been unable to attain agreement._____

_____

_____

_____

_____

_____

8. Other comments or additions to minutes.

_____

_____

_____

_____

_____

_____

_____

_____

_____

_____

_____

_____

_____

_____

Secretary to Utilization Review Committee

naires also tested knowledge about ongoing utilization review activities at the center. Finally, the utilization review chairman and other key personnel were interviewed in person at the start of the project to gain a broad overview of each center, its organization, funding sources and problems. At the close of the project, about twelve to eighteen months later depending on the center, most utilization review committee members, senior administrators, unit chiefs, and some clinicians whose clinical work had been reviewed, were interviewed to gain their impressions of the work of the committee.

ESTABLISHING A SET

Before implementing a patient care appraisal system, it is necessary to establish a general organizational climate which generates interest in and supports the initiation of such an activity. A number of influences within and outside of the institution can be identified which contribute to establishing such a set. These include the attitudes of governmental and accrediting agents, insurance companies, citizen-consumers, the administration of the center, and the availability of a working model for performing utilization review.

Governmental and Accrediting Agents.   At the time of the PURE project, Medicare, Medicaid and the Joint Commission on Hospital Accreditation all required the existence of some form of utilization review. NIMH, which provided the initial funding for many centers, had also begun to press for more documentation concerning the quality of care provided. Interestingly enough, however, these vectors of pressure were generally regarded as implicit rather than explicit, vague rather than specific, and future rather than present-oriented. Until clearer guidelines for review were promulgated and patient care appraisal became linked to reimbursement, it appeared that nothing more than perfunctory and minimal compliance was required.

As time passed, and the pressures for the systematic monitoring of patient care mounted, concern began to emerge about the possibility of standards being developed by external agencies not involved directly in patient care. Active interest in utilization review increased. Participation in the PURE Project was viewed more charitably as a way of gaining a head start in meeting these requirements. In addition, participation was made reasonably palatable when funds and technical assistance were both provided. Without this positive reinforcement from the project, indeed it is unlikely that the threat of future regulation would have produced more than a posture of watchful waiting.

Private Third-Party Payers.   Many programs are dependent upon third party reimbursement to support their patient care activities. These agents are increasingly insistent upon justification for payment, particularly where there are questions of extended duration of stay. Where so direct a link between

reimbursement and program life is maintained, efforts at creating a positive
ambiance towards the process of review are strongly reinforced. Similarly,
the absence of such pressures is reflected in the more tentative and academic
interest in the process shown by publically supported programs operating on
fixed annual budgets and returning earned revenue to a general fund.

Citizen-Consumers. The federal CMHC program places considerable emphasis upon community involvement as a mechanism for insuring
program responsiveness. The NIMH policy and standards manual for community mental health centers stipulates that centers "involve the community
in the planning, development, and operation of the program." Our anecdotal
data revealed no expressed interest in the activity of utilization review on the
part of those communities interacting with the participating centers. Members
of the community were reported to be most interested in questions related
to personnel practices, the difficulty of getting more patients into treatment,
the problem of certain patients still perceived as sick being returned so quickly
to the community, and the institution of programs felt to be more central
to the needs of the catchment areas. Such "reports" may reflect efforts to
protect peer review systems from more public scrutiny. When discussing
citizen-consumer inputs, provider respondents frequently questioned the
wisdom of "violating the integrity of the peer group" or the legality of any
attempt to move toward citizen participation in individual case review because of
confidentiality statutes. While some centers instituted special subcommittees to
solicit community opinions about patient care activities, direct community
involvement never became part of the review process at any of the participating
centers.

Administrative-Executive Constellation. As public accountability
becomes more an issue in the health and mental health fields, one may anticipate
an increase in the extrainstitutional pressures outlined above. However, the
posture of center administration towards review remains quintisential in
establishing an organizational set supportive of utilization review.

Resistance showed itself in several typical ways. The question was
asked, "Can we afford to do it?" This question suggested the existence of
competing priorities. The need to increase direct patient care and indirect
mental health services is perceived as an issue of greater urgency than assessing
the appropriateness, adequacy, effectiveness and efficiency of current activities.
Staff time, an important resource, had to be protected for service. A more
positive attitude was evidenced by making time available to reflect and evaluate.
Providing more services immediately may mean providing less in the long run.

Another manifestation of resistance was the statement: "This is
nothing new." Proponents of this view claimed that the center had many
committees, including records and information committees, medical audit

committees and service-executive committees charged with the task of monitoring patient care. Thus, considerable time was already being devoted to the task of review—albeit under differing titles. This point of view, however, was only partially true. A utilization review committee has the potential of bringing a unique point of view to questions related to the adequacy of care and the utilization of resources—that of an independent group of peers. It is well known to industrial psychologists that workers perform better if they are permitted and invited to look at the results of their work from a managerial point of view. The transition may be difficult, but it becomes impossible unless the right of independent inquiry and disagreement is sanctioned by those responsible for program administration.

Even where the posture of the administrative/executive constellation was supportive of review, overwhelming endorsement produced a backlash. Staff became suspicious of the process as a vehicle for administrative control and monitoring. Similarly, staff at times interpreted strong administrative support as evidence of a "bandwagon" effect or a temporary innovation soon to be replaced by others and, therefore, not worth the investment of time or energy. Thus, it appears inadvisable to provide more support for utilization review activities than for any other ongoing necessary function of the institution. Such evaluation activities were most successful if regarded as part of the "routine" performance of work within the center.

Availability of a Model for Utilization Review.   Whether the institution accepted or rejected the model proposed by the PURE Project, its staff had something concrete to which they could respond, bringing into focus a host of issues concerning the evaluation of patient care. In addition, the availability of specific aids such as a chart review checklist, previously validated criteria and case selection mechanisms enhanced the acceptance and furthered the performance of utilization review. It is our view that this positive response was less a reflection of the product's value per se than of the availability of something tangible and explicit in an area characterized by non-specific guidelines and procedural ambiguity.

FORMING A UTILIZATION REVIEW COMMITTEE

Committee Size and Membership

Once a favorable set was established, the task of forming a utilization review committee within the framework of governmental and accrediting regulations could begin. In general such regulations place emphasis on developing a system tailored to the needs and resources of a particular institution. There is wide latitude in the organizational formats which are satisfactory. For example, although Medicare regulations state that utilization review be conducted by a standing committee, it is possible to assign utilization review functions to an already existing committee such as medical records. In the event that the staff of a center is too small to conduct proper utilization review, assistance could be requested from an outside source.

The NIMH staff paper on utilization review suggested cross-discipline, multi-unit representation. Most centers' personnel felt that the composition of the committee should reflect the entire scope of practice within the institution. As a general rule, all disciplines primarily involved with the provision of services, clinical and non-clinical, merited consideration for membership. Since many issues raised during the course of the review relate to administrative policy, the center director or a designated surrogate usually served as a member or member ex officio. Likewise, staff responsible for record keeping and data processing were usually represented. In some centers, because of the large size and multiplicity of units, staff were invited to join the committee temporarily when specific areas of study, in which they had special competence or interest, were selected for review. Community/consumer participation was usually limited.

At all four centers, nominations for membership were received from many sources (e.g., self, service chief, UR chairman); however, the actual appointment was always made by the center director. It is of interest that at the one-year follow-up interviews the participants felt in general that the number and type of members and their mechanism of appointment were reasonable for their particular institution. Additionally, committee members felt that overlapping membership in terms of length of appointment was important. At all the centers, committee members were initially appointed for one-year terms with the understanding that some would continue beyond that time in order to allow new members joining the committee to learn from more experienced members and thus provide continuity.

At Center D the number of services made unit representation prohibitive. The center decided instead to choose a representative from all disciplines of staff not attached to particular units. This resulted in a committee whose members were at a fairly high level within the institution. Unit staffs were invited to attend the utilization review meetings as consultants when their own units were being reviewed.

At Center A, which also had many units, a different approach was taken. A small task-group discussed the details of implementing a utilization review procedure. This group was to determine the exact size and composition of the committee, select the prospective chairman and create an atmosphere in which the work of the committee would be accepted positively within the institution. The group reported that determination of the size and composition of the prospective committee could easily be accomplished by administration; they felt, however, that a more favorable climate for review would exist if there were maximal staff involvement early in the process of committee development. A major staff education campaign was begun with the gradual dissemination of information about the concept of utilization review throughout the center, a campaign which raised questions more than it provided answers. In the process, however, staff interest was generated in an issue that had previously occupied a low priority. Next, a well publicized invitation to participate in the work of the committee was extended to every staff member. Prospective members, defined by their own freely expressed interest, were then interviewed, and their ideas about peer review and self-evaluation were incorporated by the task group.

At this stage of development, it seemed important to disassociate committee functioning from the administration of the center. The concept of the peer, as opposed to the expert evaluator, was emphasized. In a large institution, where the power of administration is invariably identified with bureaucratic management of human problems, the emphasis on independence and broad representation was felt to be crucial. As a result, a committee evolved consisting of 23 members, most of whom were line staff not service chiefs, department heads or managerial personnel. Mental health workers, nurses, social workers and supportive service personnel, rather than only physicians and administrators, were on the committee.

There was a possibility that such a committee structure might generate tension within the organization through the blurring of lines of authority and accountability. To prevent this, formal links were forged to the policy-setting apparatus of the center by channeling the committee's reports of its findings and recommendations to the director (executive group) and to the clinical chiefs (service group). The intent of this linkage was to minimize the possibility of the committee developing an adversary position by insuring it access and input to the policy making mechanisms of the center.

The Committee Chairman

All participants viewed the selection of the chairman as the most tangible indication of the importance administration attached to utilization review. Whether that individual was a clinician or non-clinician tended to be a determination made on the basis of task, the level of interdisciplinary working relations, individual skill and competence and the bylaws of the institution. It is of interest to note that a psychiatrist was not designated chairman at any of the participating centers.

At Center A, the committee was chaired by a senior psychiatric social worker, assigned full time to utilization review activities. He was the only full-time chairman. In addition, he was provided with technical assistance and manpower by the center's evaluation unit. A social worker was also the chairman at Center B. Although he worked on a part-time basis, he was viewed as important since he often functioned as a trouble shooter for the center's director. Nonetheless, limitations on time occasionally affected the level of committee functioning. A psychologist was the chairman at Center C. A non-clinician, she was unable to establish rapport with the center director, a psychiatrist. Despite many fresh ideas and much enthusiasm, she ultimately resigned. The committee never felt the full impact of close support from administration. At the fourth center, the committee was also chaired by a full-time head of the evaluation unit, a clinical psychologist whose relationship to administration seemed distant. Few resource personnel were available in support of the utilization review activity.

The committee chairmen had a central role in establishing working relationships with the directors, others in administration, various standing committees and each center's unit chiefs. Their perceived power in the institutional hierarchy strongly influenced committee morale and effectiveness, and their personalities and leadership styles helped shape each committee's evolution. In one center, the chairman seemed to speak for the assistant director; and on occasion the utilization review process appeared to act as a rubber stamp to legitimize decisions already made regarding patient care. By the time the project terminated, such perceptions were beginning to seep down in the organization. One must wonder at the potential negative effect such a situation creates in relation to the acceptance of utilization review.

THE EVOLVING COMMITTEE

The Statement and Restatement of Objectives

The new committee appointed by the director of an institution initially consisted of a collection of people. They had not yet formed into a group. They did not know exactly what their task was. They did not know what was expected of them or how to act to meet these expectations. Our observations suggest the existence of two modes of committee development. One involves strict adherence to parliamentary rules, the use of a formal agenda, rigid task orientation and the specification of accountability and linkage to other structural elements within the institution. Strong emphasis upon this developmental mode corresponded with major concern on the part of committee members about issues related to status, recognition and prestige. An alternative mode of committee development involved more open processes of group formation, including the gradual clarification of issues related to natural leadership, the evolution of subgroups and factions, the establishment of internal boundaries and testing of the chairman's authority. Both modes occurred at some time in the evolution of all four committees, reflecting a committee's needs both to function within the structure of an institution and to develop a group identity and cohesiveness.

The quest for establishing a group identity at times led to a misinterpretation of a committee's objectives. There was a devaluation of the review and educative functions and a tendency to equate accomplishment with the ability to influence institutional policy. The focus on policy was supported on the basis of its providing a clearer measure of committee effectiveness and status. The impact of review on individual patient care was viewed as an ephemeral and intangible objective, far more difficult to measure than substantive changes in administrative policy. In those centers where questions related to the quality of care and program enrichment assumed lesser importance than issues of power, the committees gradually became alienated from both peers and administration.

To avoid the development of a committee-as-adversary, it was necessary for administration to restate and refine objectives repeatedly during the early evolutionary phase. Lack of a clear mandate from administration and lack of clarity about role corresponded with periods of low morale in the utilization revue committees, evidenced by a drop in attendance and a lower level of enthusiasm reported by the research assistants.

As a group of peers, the utilization review committee was expected to look at the work of colleagues and to contribute, through the review process, to an improvement in the quality and efficiency of patient care. The most justifiable and reasonable outcome measures for such a committee would be either a change in the quality of clinical care provided or maintenance of the same quality of care at a lower cost. The utilization review committee had to maintain a consistent focus upon the care provided the average patient and not upon the number of policy recommendations presented to or approved by administration.

It is of interest that while at all centers they initially set out to concentrate on improving patient care through individual case review, at two of them the committees were immediately faced with the pragmatic concern that case records were so unstandardized and incomplete as to make case review virtually impossible. Thus the first major focus of the utilization review committees was either to assume responsibility for the records and establish a record subcommittee or to prod the existing records committee into a more effective performance of its job. At another center the committee from the outset abandoned all attempts at individual case review and focused on special topics such as staffing patterns, availability of foster homes in the community, continuity of service. It was this last committee that ran into the most resistance from administration, having its chairman ultimately resign from the institution. No individual case review was ever performed, and the committee was still groping for a way to be effective by the end of the PURE Project.

The Acceptance of Role

Over time, members of the utilization review committee had to adapt to the uniqueness of their role. Since they were frequently called upon to appraise the work of clinicians more experienced than themselves or occupying positions of authority within the institution, the acceptance of role did not prove easy. Aside from individual personality factors, a number of group phenomena and institutional factors were identified which influenced role acceptance.

Individuation and Specialization within the Groups. The capability of each member to contribute by virtue of his background, experience and particular expertise had to be reinforced. A pharmacist could comfortably act as an expert when only the toxicity of drugs was discussed. However, he would not so easily raise more clinically-oriented questions about the suicidal potential of a patient, even when medication was prescribed in potentially lethal amounts. Unless individual members felt that others valued not only their specialized contributions but also their special personal qualities, they would eschew any role on the committee.

Avoidance of Potential Conflict of Interest. At none of the four centers were individual committee members involved in the investigation of care provided on units where they worked as primary clinicians. In no circumstances did the clinician who was treating the patient act as a reviewer of the case.

Legitimization. The nature of accountability in professional organizations is often quite ambiguous. It is not unusual for a service chief to view himself as an independent agent, minimally responsible to administration, especially in the area of direct clinical care. Interference with what is perceived as "strictly clinical matters" is strongly resisted. To a certain extent, all clinicians within an institution adopt a similar posture in relation to the patients for whom they are responsible. Additionally, each discipline attempts to maintain its control in relation to specialized patient care functions.

These realities make it apparent that every committee member was subjected to a host of pressures from the many reference groups to which he belonged. These pressures could not be resisted unless the role of reviewer was legitimized within the institution and the independence of the committee supported. Members would not continue to participate in a function which they felt placed them in jeopardy on their unit, among their peers or within their discipline.

Administrative Support and Positive Reinforcement. Rarely was administrative support for participation shown by relieving members of other responsibilities in order to participate in the committee's work. This was a source of dissatisfaction for most members, but was felt to be typical of the usual institutional response to a new activity. In only one center was the chairman involved full time in the review process and related activities.

The administration's response to the recommendations of the committee, however, was an important factor in influencing the members' acceptance of their role. At all centers there was a strong desire to effect change directly and a dissatisfaction with being primarily a recommending group. For example, morale on one committee continued to fall and membership to decrease until the committee chairman met with the clinical directors. In order that the UR activity would have a direct input, he was appointed as a member to this policy-making committee. At the same time, agreement was reached to allow committee members to interview clinicians directly about patient care issues arising from chart review. The former step was viewed as an acknowledgement of value and status, the latter as a demonstration of trust and respect. Membership soon stabilized and morale increased markedly.

Peer Acceptance.   The response of peers to the activities of the committee also influenced role acceptance. Peer responses are predicated upon a view of the review process as primarily educative/supportive rather than judgmental/punitive. Where committee membership was seen as inducing the metamorphosis of colleagues from peers to overseers, pressure developed on members to quit the committee. A survey conducted at all of the centers revealed a very positive response on the part of staff to peer review as an educational endeavor. Over 50 percent of the clinicians desired more review of their work.

The Establishment of Operational Procedures
Once the objectives of the utilization review activity were stated, restated and internalized, it was necessary for the committee to establish standard procedures for case selection, record review, requests for additional information and documentation of performed activities. Since many of the specific techniques have been discussed elsewhere in this volume, it will be useful at this juncture to focus on the functioning of one committee.

The members of the committee at Center A began their work with the assumption that they should not only be involved in individual case review but also explore broad issues related to the utilization of the institution. As a result, they divided the committee into three subgroups: a Statistical Analysis and Review Subcommittee, a Consumer Opinion Subcommittee and a Patient Care Subcommittee.

The Statistical Analysis and Review Subcommittee was involved with the analysis of aggregate data on admissions, readmissions, length of treatment, etc. Much of these data were easily available because of the computerized MSIS record system. To gain a firmer understanding of the magnitude and complexity of the center's work and to identify gaps and deficiencies in service, the subcommittee also undertook the analysis of patterns of care and special studies. For example, they studied the number of walk-in patients and no-show patients to the assessment and brief-treatment unit of the center. They documented that an increase in the no-show rate was a corollary of an increase in the delay between initial contact and subsequent contacts with the center. Various recommendations were made in regard to streamlining admission forms and modifying admission procedure. These results were forwarded to administration and implemented.

The Consumer Opinion Subcommittee independently investigated clients opinions about care and analyzed complaints of referring institutions and practitioners. Not only did their work help in selecting individual cases for review and focus attention on problem areas in the institution, but their efforts helped to address areas in which consumer dissatisfaction could be turned into criteria for adequate care.

The Patient Care Subcommittee worked in conjunction with an evaluation unit which performed the three-stage review on those charts selected either randomly or on the basis of defined topical issues that were felt by the URC to merit detailed study. Each month the evaluation unit generated a report which included a synopsis of each chart that had been reviewed. Below is an example of one case from such a report:

> This is the chart of a 26-year-old, white, single female who was unemployed and lived alone at admission. This was the sixth CMHC admission for Y whose prior psychiatric history included multiple hospitalizations at other treatment facilities. Her diagnosis was schizophrenia, paranoid type, and she was referred from the emergency room in an actively psychotic state. At the time of admission, she was noted to be very ambivalent about hospitalization; although she signed the voluntary admission form, she said she did not need hospitalization and continued to express this. After three weeks on the unit, in which she showed minimal involvement with the community, she went AWOL while on buddy status. The patient's mother was notified and the patient was discharged AMA [against medical advice] with a note in the chart that she was to be readmitted if she came back to the unit at a later date. At Level II review, the chart was found deficient in Assessment for Suicide and because the patient left AMA. The clinical consultant noted that suicidal behavior should be addressed more completely in the data base. He also noted that, despite the fact that the patient was an extremely difficult management problem who was well known to the unit, it was not clear that the treatment team had a clear understanding or formulation of the patient's behavior; given her history, some restrictions should have been placed on her leaving the ward. He felt there was an inconsistent policy about sanctions on the patient for leaving "group meetings" or accepting treatment recommendations. The consultant felt that the chart was inadequate with respect both to adequacy of recording and of care. He noted that there was no integrated use of past work-ups to arrive at an understanding of the dynamics. He noted also that there was a failure of rigorous follow-up after the patient left AMA. The consultant suggests that, given the patient's history, more attempts, [such] as alerting police, 15-day paper, and home visits, should have been made. He felt that the deficiencies in recording and care could be handled by getting in touch with the

clinicians and supervisors but raises the issue for the URC of the center's clinical and legal responsibilities for follow-up of AMAs.

Upon receipt of reports such as this one, subcommittee members were free to augment the data through further review of the charts, meeting with the involved clinicians and/or supervisors or consultation with center staff felt to be expert in the area being considered. Once the data from the review, report, interviews with clinicians, and expert opinion had been collated and discussed in the subcommittee, decisions related to further action were made. In this case example, the subcommittee contacted the clinicians to discuss the consultants' observations (after securing approval from the entire utilization review committee). In addition this case raised the issue of the lack of any institutional guidelines concerning the treatment of patients who leave AMA (against medical advice).

The subcommittee decided to select a sample of patients who had been discharged AMA during a three-month period in order to help answer the following questions:

> What should the clinical responsibility of the center be for follow-up of patients who leave AMA? What are legal responsibilities? When should the police be notified? When are home visits appropriate? Should the AMA category be used for outpatients as well as in-patients? Should the AMA category be reserved for only patients in life-threatening situations? Should a physician be required to sign a note when the patient leaves AMA? Should a physician be required to countersign the discharge summary of a patient who leaves AMA?

Thus the subcommittee began an investigation of the problem of the AMA patient and ultimately formulated several suggestions as to changes in the record system, changes in criteria for follow-up care, and clarification of the physician's role in treatment. These recommendations, as well as comments about individual cases, were forwarded to the URC as a whole. The URC then sent its recommendations to the appropriate policy setting group in the center who responded by accepting some of them and implementing appropriate changes.

Not only did the patient care subcommittee contact clinicians whose work was deficient, but on occasion, when care was excellent, the clinician would also be notified. In dealing with clinicians the subcommittee members were careful to emphasize the educative and informative rather than the censuring or punitive aspect of the review. Interviews with these clinicians indicated satisfaction with the reviewers' efforts.

In Center A the various subcommittees met bi-monthly; the entire utilization review committee met on a monthly basis. Complete minutes were taken. Reports from the various subcommittees were reviewed and appropriate action taken. As the example above indicates, these actions ranged from approval to contact clinicians or supervisors, to recommending changes in the record keeping system, to changes in criteria, to suggesting to administration certain policy changes.

CONCLUSION

In the past, the division of labor for monitoring patient care has taken various forms depending upon the organizational structure, goals and resources of an institution. In some instances, a single unit was designated as responsible for patient care evaluation; in others, separate groups were responsible for medical audit, patient records, and admission procedures. It was not until the beginning of the Medicare program, that institutions were required, as a condition of participation, to make a commitment to a course of action in patient care surveillance and file a written description of their proposed utilization review program.

While Medicare standards for utilization review are flexible and encourage experimentation, they call for the following:

—A written plan describing the structural and functional aspects of the review program, approved by the staff and governing body;
—A two-stage process involving (a) a review of admissions, duration of stays and professional services furnished, on a sample of other basis, ". . . with respect to the necessity of the services and for the purpose of promoting the most efficient use of available facilities and services. Such reviews are to emphasize identification and analysis of patient care in order to maintain high quality," and (b) a review of each case of extended duration, defined by the medical staff itself;
—The conduct of the utilization review function by a committee (or committees) internal or external to the hospital, either established for the unique function of utilization review or for some other purpose, but able to execute the above requirements.
—A record of committee activities with periodic reports to the entire medical staff and governing body of the hospital; and;
—Evidence of staff support for committee function and assistance to attending staff in making the most appropriate use of available facilities and services.

Thus, the Medicare law merely requires that utilization review be performed; the regulations simply detailed the types of activities required. The actual performance is left entirely to the institution or agency, its utilization review committee, and supporting staff. State health department personnel, responsible for monitoring compliance by institutions, seek only to ascertain that utilization review is actually being performed, not to question any decisions or recommendations made by the utilization review committee.

Careful review of conditions of participation and their official interpretation reveals an emphasis upon insuring appropriate quality that is entirely consistent with recommendations made by various professional organizations in the past. In a sense, the Medicare formulation represents an operational translation of the professional communities' existent concern for providing more effective and efficient service.

Since the applicability of the regulations is limited to the review of Medicare beneficiaries' hospitalization, the Medicare conditions are included primarily for illustrative purposes. In point of fact, as other agencies and insurors become concerned with the quality of service rendered to their clients, an expansion of utilization review's scope can easily be envisioned. Indeed, public Law 92-603 has recently made provision for federal monitoring of patient care evaluation through the establishment of the Professional Standards Review Organization (PSRO). The PSRO provision created a nationwide network of locally based physician groups for reviewing the necessity, and quality of health services covered under Medicare and Medicaid and provided in hospitals and nursing homes. Initially, PSRO activities will be focused upon institutional care. With HEW approval, however, they could assume responsibility in relation to non-institutional care. The legislation speaks explicitly to the development of norms and the use of criteria in evaluating patient care as well as the analysis of aggregate data for reviewing profiles of care and the services rendered to patients. Current hospital utilization review committees are not invalidated. The law requires the PSRO's acknowledge and accept, in part or wholly, an institution's internal review where such review committee's demonstrate effective quality and utilization controls.

Clearly, the growing public subsidy of medical care has led to a merger of the principle of quality assurance with that of public accountability. As a result, it is imperative that professional review mechanisms such as Utilization Review not only be technically correct but also effective. For that to occur, however, attention must be paid not only to technique but also to a host of psychosocial and organizational factors that may alternate the effectiveness of patient care appraisal. With this in mind, we have devoted the present chapter to the consideration of the institutional context within which patient care appraisal unfolds.

The chapter has touched upon a number of issues affecting the establishment of on-going utilization review activity in community mental health centers. Specific attention has been focused on (1) the need for certain extrainstitution supports (guidelines, funding, technical resources), (2) intra-institutional supports (administrative interest and allocation of resources), (3) effect of group phenomena (establishing trust, cohesiveness, identity),

(4) effect of individual adaptation to the role of a non-authoritarian, peer-teacher, and finally (5) the need for adequate feedback mechanisms to foster change.

In summary, a well-conducted utilization review activity enhances other methods of program evaluation in mental health. The use of predetermined criteria for case selection and case review provides an objective standard with which to measure the quality of care rendered during treatment. This dimension of evaluation relates to the overall goal of the institution to deliver the highest feasible quality of patient care to those it is mandated to serve. In addition, the analyses of patterns of care not only contribute to the further refinement of criteria for selection and review but also provide the necessary data to assess whether program goals are being met. For example, are waiting lists shorter? more alcoholics being treated? or is the drug program reaching the designated target population? In brief, while meeting the requirements of Medicare and the Joint Committee on Accreditation, utilization review can also become an integral part of an institution's program evaluation activities.

The continued effectiveness of a utilization review committee relies heavily upon the maintenance of open channels of communication. Through these channels will flow a wide variety of information: facts, recommendations, conclusions, hypotheses, consumer complaints, administrative directives and an assortment of other items. If channels clog, then staff interest and investment in the utilization review process will atrophy. Eventually the committee will cease to exist except on paper. Since the variety of organizational configurations within mental health centers precludes the possibility of prescribing specific antidotes to this problem, we can only indicate that communication and feedback are essential to the survival of an effective utilization review committee.

The process of review itself offers an institution the opportunity and provides it the blueprint for meaningful self-evaluation. One natural by-product of the process is a heightened concern for quality of care, a concern whose potential benefits exceed the value of any report to a regulatory or fiduciary agency. Other benefits to be derived from the process of utilization review include an increased awareness on the part of staff members of the effects their practices have on center costs and utilization problems. The interaction between clinical staff and administration centering around the task of utilization review, provides an excellent opportunity for increased understanding and rapport between the two groups. The experience and educational aspects of utilization review should not only result in a higher quality of patient care but also raise substantive questions related to such issues as accessibility and public accountability. Greater concern for justified admissions, an early product of utilization review, leads to the expansion of services available in an outpatient or outreach setting. Also, an increased institutionalized concern for reducing lengths of stay may enable the center to offer its services to a greater number of patients.

The optimal result of utilization review can easily be described in terms of basic health economics: to provide a scarce service of the highest quality to the largest possible population at a reasonable cost.

Suggested Guidelines for Establishing a Utilization Review Committee

I. THE SIZE AND COMPOSITION OF THE COMMITTEE

While the Joint Committee on Accreditation merely stipulates that a review process must exist, Medicare regulations state that utilization review should be conducted by a standing committee. Since the preexistent review functions of records review and medical audit overlap to some degree with utilization review, it is possible to assign the utilization review function to one or more of a facility's standing committees. If the staff of a facility is too small to conduct all aspects of utilization review, assistance may be requested from an outside source. With the approval of the governing authority it is possible to retain any outside consultants.

The actual number of committee members should, at least, conform to Medicare regulations and should be determined by the size and organization of the center, the task of the committee and the breadth of the program. The composition of the committee should reflect the entire scope of practice within the facility. As a general rule, the committee should have representation from all disciplines primarily involved in the provision of service, clinical and non-clinical.

Since many issues raised during the course of review will be related to administrative policy, the director (or his designated surrogate) and staff responsible for record keeping and data processing should serve as members or members ex officio. When specific areas of study are selected in which the committee members lack a specific competence, other staff representatives should be invited to serve on a temporary basis.

Many mental health centers have learned that their utilization review functions are expedited through the formation of permanent sub-committees. The focal point of each subcommittee should be consistent with the professional background, interest, or skills of its members. Thus, a medical record librarian would naturally serve on the subcommittee on records and data. All subcommittees should meet at least monthly, and their proceedings and recommendations should be incorporated as a standing item on the agenda of the parent utilization review committee. Mental health centers may institute one or more of the following subcommittee types:

A. Records and Data.   This subcommittee monitors the quality of patient care documentation and reporting within the center. The quality and quantity of statistics and reports generated for or within the center are regularly reviewed by this group. Membership of this subcommittee should include the center's medical record librarian and its statistician or director of electronic data processing.

B. Consumer Subcommittee.   This subcommittee can serve as a patient complaint review board. All consumer complaints should be directed to this group for a timely review of the complaint and response to the consumer. This group can collectively act as an investigative body as well as perform an important function for the parent committee. The subcommittee on consumer complaints can report monthly to the utilization review committee regarding the perceived and reported reactions of consumers to the institution's staff, policy and practices.

C. Patient Care Subcommittee.   This subcommittee should serve as a means of specifically looking at individual cases to determine if the care described at least meets minimal acceptable standards.

D. Special Studies.   Experience indicates that the activities of utilization review necessitate or indicate the need for special studies to be conducted within the institution. Frequently, these studies can be conducted by members of the center staff, as in a review of frequency-by-diagnostic admissions to different components of the center.

II. APPOINTMENT OF MEMBERS

Appointment of the chairman and committee members should be made in accordance with the existing bylaws of the center. The committee members should have both the skills and interest to serve. The selection of the chairman should reflect the fact that utilization review is an important task. Depending upon the scope of utilization review activities within a given institution and the nature of interdisciplinary working relationships, the position can be filled by a clinician or non-clinician.

Since it takes a fair amount of time to establish working relationships and to become familiar with utilization review techniques, the term of appointment should be for more than one year. To provide continuity, only a portion of the membership should change each year. For example, members could be appointed for three-year terms, with one third of the members changing each year. However, at times it may be useful to establish special committees, chaired by members of the utilization review committee, which include other members of the center appointed specially for a particular task.

Membership should not be determined solely on the basis of authority or experience. Since the committee will scrutinize the work of both administrative units and individuals, representation should be open to staff at all levels, (e.g., the psychiatrist-in-chief, the director of outpatient services, a resident in training, a community health worker).

III. MEETINGS

The utilization review committee should meet as a group at least once a month, keeping a permanent record of the proceedings. More frequent meetings may be held if necessary. While assignments may be given to subcommittees or individual committee members, the final responsibility for review and recommendation rests with the committee as a whole.

IV. LIAISON RELATIONSHIPS

A utilization review committee should maintain liaison relationships with:

A. The director of the center. The support of administration facilitates the conduct of studies necessary to highlight areas and practices which influence utilization. In addition, the director has to approve changes in organizational patterns or administrative procedures to improve utilization patterns.

B. The records committee. Since the work of utilization review committee is largely dependent upon the availability of up-to-date records which contain sufficient information to permit both decisions and objective review, participation of representatives from the record committee is essential. The analyses of the utilization review committee may point up inadequacies in charts and lead to recommendations for improvement of records.

C. The executive officers of the center. This group, which may include heads of different units, representatives from different disciplines and members of the community, is responsible for defining the broad policy and mission of a facility and needs to know about the efficiency and effectiveness of its program. Reports that contain the manner of selection, statistical findings, analysis of findings, trends and their significance and pertinent recommendations for action should be made regularly to the executive committee.

V. COMMITTEE TASKS

A. Individual Case Review.   In general, the committee will review and evaluate both retrospectively and concurrently, patient records including extended duration. Concurrent analysis allows for modification of care while the individual is still receiving service. Retrospective analysis focuses on generating information about what happened in the past and is, therefore, generally less threatening to staff. Concurrent analysis is more effectively done when criteria defining deviant care have been normatively developed by clinical panels and when pattern analysis has been used in retrospective case review.

The number of charts to be reviewed is a function of the size of the center, the number of members serving on the committee or the number of staff assigned to case review. Charts should be read in advance, and participants should be prepared to discuss them at scheduled meetings. To the extent possible, each committee member should review, based on experience and training, those cases in which his judgment would be best.

When examining charts, a checklist or review form lends consistency to the review process. The checklist should be comprehensive enough to provide an adequate view of the patient yet restricted to information pertinent and necessary to the review. To keep records confidential, the patient should be identified by hospital number and service unit only.

B. The Selection of Cases.   The manner in which a committee selects areas of concentration depends upon the sources of data available and the technical level of data processing. The use of automated screening processes for case selection is highly advisable. Such a method allows purposive selection of cases that deviate from expected patterns of care and that are of special interest to the committee and permits random sampling of the remainder of the patient population.

C. Obtaining of Additional Information.   Committee members should be encouraged to seek out involved staff. A general policy on the conditions under which such information is solicited and the manner in which it is done should be developed. Further, the committee can direct special studies, such as determining various utilization rates of the center by groups in the community. Or the committee can undertake brief outcome studies to verify the utility of services and validate criteria.

D. Documentation.   The utilization committee should maintain adequate records summarizing its activities. Summaries can be developed from data reported by committee members and incorporated as part of the committee's minutes. All utilization review committee records, including the review form or checklist, should be kept confidential and not be filed with individuals' medical records.

E. Modification of Clinical Practice. An important function of utilization review activities is to feed back information from the review process to the clinical staff providing day-to-day patient care. In order to achieve the institution's goals of providing high quality patient care, findings from pattern analysis or case review may demand changes in clinical practices or suggest closer scrutiny of the functioning of a single clinician or group of clinicians. For example, the occurrence of suicides after discharge from a crisis intervention unit may indicate the need for a more thorough routine clinical evaluation at termination of treatment, with provision for extended duration of inpatient stay when it is indicated by a high potential for suicide on the mental status examination. In some cases questioning of the individual clinician responsible for the early discharge of a patient who later suicided will be warranted.

To be sure, it is easier in some ways to effect a change in administrative policy than to confront a clinician with some deficiencies in patient care. Within most care giving institutions, modes are already established for bringing about changes in policy. On the other hand, critical review of the work of the individual clinician by a review committee is an activity for which there is no uniformly established feedback mechanism. In many institutions, clinicians at certain levels, particularly those in training, are supervised by senior staff members. Information feedback, then, can be routed through the supervisors. However, in some institutions, particularly those without a training component, supervision of clinical staff may be minimal. In such instances it will be particularly important to carefully consider ways of feeding back information from the review process to effect changes in clinical practice without unnecessarily threatening the autonomy or security of the treating clinician.

F. Modification of the Review Process. The findings generated by pattern analysis and case review should be routinely employed by the utilization review committee to assess the adequacy of both its selection mechanisms and the criteria used in the evaluation of the quality of patient care. A sensitive review process should always reflect the best contemporary statement of appropriate patterns of treatment.

Appendix A

Members of PURE Project

Principal Investigator
D. Riedel

Co-principal Investigators
H. Brenner
G. Klerman
J. Myers
G. Tischler

Research Associates
L. Brauer
P. Goldblatt
F. Greaney
R. Morisse
C. Schwartz

Data Group
H. Brenner (Chairman)
L. Brauer (Liaison with CMHC and Panels)
P. Goldblatt (Liaison with CMHC and Panels)
A. Lerman
M. Levine
S. Markowitz
C. Stancliff
J. Vitale
P. Walker
S. Wyde

also Coders and Keypunch Operators

243

Intake Panel
  S. Kasl (Chairman)
  H. Flynn
  V. Garrison
  J. Henisz
  M. Levine
  H. Zonana
  L. Brauer (Liaison)

Suicide Panel
  E. Paykel (Chairman)
  D. Dressler
  N. French
  C. Hallowell
  H. Mark
  D. Shapiro
  R. Steele
  M. Weissman
  A. Ward
  P. Goldblatt (Liaison)

Adolescent Panel
  L. Zegans (Chairman)
  H. Flynn
  J. Geller
  J. Schowalter
  M. Sullivan
  M. Swartzburg
  P. Goldblatt (Liaison)

Schizophrenia Panel
  B. Astrachan (Chairman)
  M. Harrow
  A. Schwartz
  G. Tucker
  L. Brauer (Liaison)

Schizophrenia Field Study
  J. Myers (Chairman)
  B. Astrachan
  H. Brenner
  L. Brauer (Liaison)
  C. Schwartz

Outpatient Field Study
  H. Zonana (Chairman)
  R. Berberian

G. Klerman
B. Prusoff
G. Tischler
P. Goldblatt (Liaison)

Epidemiological Survey
J. Henisz
G. Tischler
J. Myers

Research Assistants
D. Adler
M. Bart
B. Bosma
P. Boswell
G. Brown
C. Cappello
W. Daley
M. Davis
K. Fox
B. Goldberg
P. Jeffers
P. Krauss
M. Malcolm-Lawes
B. Mostue
P. Newberry
L. Royen
B. Smith
M. Snyder

Programmers
R. Averill
M. Condry
J. Cunningham
A. Docherty
E. Elia
W. Leng
L. Mills
P. Walker

Secretaries
A. Leonardo
M. Milner

Editorial Assistant
D. Cesaroni

Appendix B

Checklist for Direct Patient Care Evaluation

INTRODUCTION

This checklist is a modification and expansion of an "Admissions/Intake Checklist (Revision 1)" developed by the Psychiatric Utilization Review and Evaluation (PURE) Project at Yale University. The PURE Project checklist consisted of a compilation of criteria about adequacy of the intake/evaluation as recorded in a chart. Those criteria were developed by four peer group panels of clinicians meeting over a period of two years. The panels, made up of psychiatrists, psychologists, nurses, social workers and social scientists, worked in four areas: schizophrenia, suicide, adolescence, and intake. These areas were selected for experimental reasons as described in the PURE Project manual.[a] The PURE Project checklist was then modified by the Program Information and Analysis Section (PIAS) of the Connecticut Mental Health Center (CMHC) to conform to the needs of the CMHC chart review procedures and to include criteria of treatment, as well as intake evaluation, and criteria in several areas not included in the PURE Project checklist. The criteria which are being added to the checklist by the PIAS unit are drawn in large part from the work of the PURE Project panels which went beyond the intake and evaluation process included in the original checklist. These additional criteria, particularly in the area of treatment, must be considered at this point in time, merely suggestions for inclusion. Before this checklist is implemented for Utilization Review at the CMHC, it will be submitted to a panel or panels of experts to review the additional criteria and arrive at a consensus as to the standards of care to be reflected in review.

The utilization review process in the CMHC will be accomplished in three successive stages, or levels of review, which will differ in the number of .

[a]Donald C. Riedel, Principal Investigator, "Guidelines for Psychiatric Utilization Review in Community Mental Health Centers," Vol. 1, Progress Report No. 4, Jan., 1971–July, 1971, Contract HSM-42-69-60, National Institute of Mental Health.

charts reviewed, the expertise with which review will be accomplished and the extent and quality of information reviewed. The three levels of review are reflected in the format of the checklist. The first level review, contained on the first two pages of the checklist, will be applied to charts on all patients admitted to treatment at the CMHC and will be accomplished by Records Room personnel. The goal of this level of review is to establish the completeness of the information contained in the charts. Charts which are found to not meet the minimal standards of completeness as required by the checklist will be returned to the attending clinician for completion.

The second level review (Column 1, pp. 3, "PIAS Review") will be accomplished on samples of charts selected for intensive review. PIAS Review will be accomplished by professional non-clinical personnel of the PIAS unit under the supervision of a psychiatrist. The basis on which charts will be selected for intensive review remains to be established, but will follow guidelines and suggestions made by the PURE Project panels. The goals of this level of review are to: (1) establish the adequacy of the information contained in the chart for clinical review and (2) establish whether or not the treatment reflected in the information included in the chart meets the criteria of good patient care set forth in the checklist. This level review is not intended to establish adequacy of clinical care but only conformity to model standards of care represented in the criteria. Judgment of adequacy of care is the function of clinical level review.

The third level review (Column 2, pp. 3ff, "Clinical Review") will be accomplished on all charts found in the PIAS review to not conform to the criteria incorporated in the checklist and on a certain proportion of charts randomly selected from those reviewed by PIAS by expert clinicians of the CMHC Utilization Review Committee. The goals of this level of review are to: (1) establish the adequacy of the patient care provided in those instances where the standards prescribed in the checklist were not followed and (2) provide continuing test of the adequacy of the criteria in the checklist to discriminate adequate and inadequate patient care at the PIAS level of review.

PRELIMINARY INSTRUCTIONS TO REVIEWERS*

A manual of instructions and definitions for standardization of use of the Chart Review Checklist is in preparation and will be completed when the Checklist is considered to be in final form. Meanwhile, there are a few conventions which have been agreed upon which should be called to the attention of reviewers employing the checklist prior to the publication of the Manual.

First, the checklist is designed to cover the latest treatment episode only. That is, if the patient has been admitted, discharged, and readmitted on

*If the patient was seen in the Evaluation Unit (100) *only* and was discharged within 4 visits or 45 days, second level review using this standard PIAS checklist should *not* be performed. A checklist for such charts is being developed.

one or more occasions, the reviewer should consider only the last admission. Information contained in the chart for prior admissions should be considered only when a note in the chart at the last admission makes explicit reference to the prior material.

Secondly, all items inquiring about the presence of information in the chart regarding symptoms or behavior manifested refer to the presence of the symptoms or the behavior during the seven days immediately preceding the evaluation only, unless otherwise specified, i.e. "a history of. . . ."

Third, the PIAS and Clinical Level Reviews assume that the chart is complete, as evidenced at the Records Room Level Review. Information in the chart should, therefore, be complete enough to make decisions on all items in the PIAS and Clinical Level Reviews. Therefore, "no information," blanks, or "not applicable," are not acceptable responses except where a reviewer is instructed to skip a section on the basis of criteria included in the checklist, or a "not applicable" (NA) category has been provided for coding and is defined by the item.

Finally, in order to provide continuing feedback for assessment and, where necessary, revision of the review criteria, the clinical reviewer is asked in all cases to explain the basis of his judgment on clinical review. Clinical reviewers are asked to please provide these explanations systematically and completely until a standard form of the checklist is developed, at which time provision will be made for an overall assessment in a more economical manner. If there is insufficient space on the face of the form to complete your explanation adequately, use the reverse side of the page.

CHART REVIEW CHECKLIST   Revised Dec., 1973

Level 1—Records Room Review[1]

I.   *Identification*   Chart Number: _____

      Patient's initials: _____   First CMHC Admission: Yes   No
      Sex:____ Birthdate:_____ Race:____   Date of Admission Reviewed:_____
      Reviewer's Name: _____   Unit of Intake: _____
      Date of Review: _____   Unit(s) on which treated: _____

                                                _____

II.   *Format of Chart*

      A. (APPLICABLE TO ALL PATIENTS) The following forms are required in all CMHC patients' charts with the exceptions indicated. Are they present and *completed* in this chart as required?
      *1. MSIS Admission Form   Yes   No

1. Note time review began and all interruptions so that time to complete review can be recorded, page 251.

   2. CMHC Supplemental Form   Yes   No

   3. Initial Contact—Referral Form *or* E.R. Sheet *or* Admission Note (inpatients admitted directly) *or* Transfer Summary from another institution dated not more than 30 days before admission to the Center. (West Haven HRC Assessment, Planning and Treatment Form substitutes for Initial Contact Form)   Yes   No

*4. PER-C or MSER (*Not* required if outpatient is discharged from Evaluation Unit (100) with or without referral, *outside* CMHC, *within* 4 sessions or 45 days)   Yes   No   NA

*5. Dictated Admission/Transfer/Discharge Summary (optional if patient is discharged from assessment (Unit 100) within 4 sessions or 45 days)   Yes   No   NA

     If YES, was it dictated within 30 days of initial visit?   Yes   No   NA

     *a. Is Admission Diagnosis recorded?   Yes   No

     *b. Is Discharge Diagnosis recorded? (If patient was at the Center less than 30 days, one diagnosis can be considered as both admission *and* discharge diagnosis)   Yes   No

     c. If the patient was treated more than 45 days *or* treated in other than Evaluation Unit (100) are there both Admission/Transfer *and* Discharge Summaries in the chart?   Yes   No   NA

   6. CMHC Change of Status Form indicating unit to which patient was first assigned (if patient admitted to treatment at CMHC)   Yes   No   NA

   7. Progress Notes (if patient is inpatient or was seen more than 30 days in an outpatient unit)   Yes   No   NA

B. (APPLICABLE TO OUTPATIENTS ONLY) Was an Outpatient Index Card maintained?   Yes   No   NA

   IF PATIENT TREATED AS OUTPATIENT ONLY, SKIP TO SECTION III.

C. (APPLICABLE TO INPATIENTS ONLY) Are the following forms present and *completed* in this chart?

   *1. MSER (if patient stayed on service more than five days) or PER-C (if patient stayed on service less than five days) (On 4th floor (111), PER is required)   Yes   No   NA / Yes   No

   2. Physical Examination Form   Yes   No

     IF YES, does chart indicate it was completed within 24 hours of admission?   Yes   No   NA

   3. Application for Admission to inpatient unit or Permission to Treat a Minor   Yes   No

   4. Doctors' Orders   Yes   No

   5. Medication Record   Yes   No   NA

III. *Disposition of Chart* (APPLICABLE TO ALL PATIENTS)

A. Is any *asterisked* item under Section II above answered No?   Yes   No
   IF YES, CHART SHOULD BE RETURNED TO CLINICIAN FOR COMPLETION.
   IF NO, RECORD ROOM REVIEW TERMINATES HERE.

B. Was the chart returned to the clinician for completion?   Yes   No   NA
   IF YES, Date of return to clinician: _____

      Date of return to Record Room: _____

C. Has the missing information been completed?   Yes   No   NA

Time required to complete Level I Review: _____

Levels 2 and 3—PIAS[1] and Clinical Reviews

	PIAS Review	Clinical Review
I. *Identification for Intensive Review*		
Basis of Selection for Review:		
Reviewer's Name:		
Reviewer's Discipline:		
Date of Review:		
Name of Intake Clinician:		XXXXXXXXXX
Supervisor's Name, if appropriate:		XXXXXXXXXX
Treating Clinician(s):		XXXXXXXXXX
Discipline of Treating Clinician(s):		XXXXXXXXXX
Supervisor(s)' Names, if appropriate:		XXXXXXXXXX

II. *Adequacy of Intake/Evaluation* — XXXXXXXXXX

A. *Referral Information and Contacts* — XXXXXXXXXX

   1. Was source of referral clearly stated?   [8]Yes_1 No_0 XXXXXXXXXX XXXXXXXXXX

   IF NO, SKIP TO ITEM II.B.   XXXXXXXXXX

   2. IF YES, should referral source have been contacted? (when referral is other than ER, self, friend, or other patient)   [9]Yes_1 No_0 NA_9 XXXXXXXXXX XXXXXXXXXX XXXXXXXXXX XXXXXXXXXX

   IF YES, was referral source contacted or, if not, was an explanation given?   [10]Yes_1 No_0 NA_9 XXXXXXXXXX XXXXXXXXXX

B. *History of Previous Treatment outside CMHC*   XXXXXXXXXX XXXXXXXXXX

   1. Is chart clear whether patient has or has not had previous treatment outside CMHC?   [11]Yes_1 No_0 XXXXXXXXXX XXXXXXXXXX XXXXXXXXXX

   IF NO, SKIP TO ITEM II.C.   XXXXXXXXXX

   2. IF YES, was patient treated previously outside CMHC?   [12]Yes_1 No_0 XXXXXXXXXX XXXXXXXXXX

   IF NO, SKIP TO ITEM II.C.   XXXXXXXXXX

   3. IF YES, were the following recorded: XXXXXXXXXX XXXXXXXXXX

     a. approximate dates   [13]Yes_1 No_0 XXXXXXXXXX

     b. facilities or clinicians names   [14]Yes_1 No_0 XXXXXXXXXX

     c. treatment modalities   [15]Yes_1 No_0 XXXXXXXXXX

---

1. Remember: Note time review began and all interruptions so that time to complete Level 2 review can be recorded on page 274.

4. Were appropriate releases obtained? ^{16}Yes$_1$ No$_0$

5. Was clinician or institution contacted or, if not, an explanation
given? ^{17}Yes$_1$ No$_0$

XXXXXXXXXX
XXXXXXXXXX
XXXXXXXXXX
XXXXXXXXXX

C. *Present Illness*

1. Is chief complaint present in
patient's own words? ^{18}Yes$_1$ No$_0$
IF NO, is it in a form which
clearly distinguishes clinician's
perception of the problem from
patient's? ^{19}Yes$_1$ No$_0$ NA$_9$

2. Is it clear why patient came? (i.e.
symptoms, changes in feelings) ^{20}Yes$_1$ No$_0$

3. Is the absence of precipitants or
the nature of the precipitants
clearly presented? ^{21}Yes$_1$ No$_0$

4. Is the chronology of the difficulty clear? ^{22}Yes$_1$ No$_0$

XXXXXXXXXX
XXXXXXXXXX
XXXXXXXXXX
XXXXXXXXXX
XXXXXXXXXX
XXXXXXXXXX
XXXXXXXXXX
XXXXXXXXXX
XXXXXXXXXX
XXXXXXXXXX
XXXXXXXXXX
XXXXXXXXXX
XXXXXXXXXX
XXXXXXXXXX
XXXXXXXXXX

D. *Drug and Alcohol Abuse*

1. Does the chart indicate that current or past history of *drug* abuse
was checked for? ^{23}Yes$_1$ No$_0$

2. Does the chart indicate that current or past history of *alcohol*
abuse was checked for? ^{24}Yes$_1$ No$_0$

IF NO TO BOTH ITEMS D. 1-2,
SKIP TO ITEM II.E.

3. IF THE CHART INDICATES A
CURRENT OR PAST HISTORY
OF DRUG OR ALCOHOL
ABUSE WAS PRESENT, were the
following indicated in the chart:
a. drug(s) used ^{25}Yes$_1$ No$_0$ NA$_9$
b. frequency of use ^{26}Yes$_1$ No$_0$ NA$_9$
c. effects ^{27}Yes$_1$ No$_0$ NA$_9$

XXXXXXXXXX
XXXXXXXXXX
XXXXXXXXXX
XXXXXXXXXX
XXXXXXXXXX
XXXXXXXXXX
XXXXXXXXXX
XXXXXXXXXX
XXXXXXXXXX
XXXXXXXXXX
XXXXXXXXXX
XXXXXXXXXX
XXXXXXXXXX
XXXXXXXXXX
XXXXXXXXXX
XXXXXXXXXX

E. *Mental Status Examination*

1. Were the following indicated on
MSER, PER-C or Admission Note:
a. appearance ^{28}Yes$_1$ No$_0$
b. attitude ^{29}Yes$_1$ No$_0$
c. mood (affect) ^{30}Yes$_1$ No$_0$
d. content and quality of speech
and thought ^{31}Yes$_1$ No$_0$
e. sensorium (sensory, orientation) ^{32}Yes$_1$ No$_0$
f. judgment ^{33}Yes$_1$ No$_0$

2. Was there a statement indicating
the overall severity of the
patient's difficulty? ^{34}Yes$_1$ No$_0$

XXXXXXXXXX
XXXXXXXXXX
XXXXXXXXXX
XXXXXXXXXX
XXXXXXXXXX
XXXXXXXXXX
XXXXXXXXXX
XXXXXXXXXX
XXXXXXXXXX
XXXXXXXXXX
XXXXXXXXXX
XXXXXXXXXX
XXXXXXXXXX

F. *Diagnosis of Schizophrenia*

1. Does the mental status examination indicate the presence of any
of the following symptoms (See
MSER or PER-C):

XXXXXXXXXX
XXXXXXXXXX
XXXXXXXXXX
XXXXXXXXXX
XXXXXXXXXX

   a. Delusions   [35] Yes_1 No_0 XXXXXXXXXX

   b. Hallucinations   [36] Yes_1 No_0 XXXXXXXXXX

   c. Bizarre thinking   [37] Yes_1 No_0 XXXXXXXXXX

   d. Looseness of associations   [38] Yes_1 No_0 XXXXXXXXXX

   e. Withdrawn   [39] Yes_1 No_0 XXXXXXXXXX

2. Does patient have a chart diagnosis of schizophrenia (APA 295.0– 295.99)   [40] Yes_1 No_0 XXXXXXXXXX

IF YES TO ANY ITEM 1–2, THE SCHIZOPHRENIC INDEX (p. 254) SHOULD BE COMPLETED. Is the Schizophrenic Index applicable?   [41] Yes_1 No_0 XXXXXXXXXX

IF NO, MARK NA IN CLINICAL REVIEW SECTIONS ITEMS F.4. AND 5., AND SKIP TO SECTION G, p. 255.

IF YES, COMPLETE SCHIZOPHRENIC INDEX, p. 254., AND RETURN TO ITEM 3.

3. Does patient have an SI score of less than 4 and a diagnosis other than schizophrenia?   [42] Yes_1 No_0 XXXXXXXXXX

IF YES, MARK NA IN CLINICAL REVIEW SECTIONS ITEMS F.4, 5 AND 6.; AND SKIP TO SECTION G, p. 255.

IF NO:

4. Does patient have an SI score of 4 or more and a diagnosis of schizophrenia?   [43] Yes_1 No_0 XXXXXXXXXX

IF YES, were the following items addressed in the chart:

   a. family history of mental illness   [44] Yes_1 No_0 NA_9 XXXXXXXXXX

   b. onset of illness in detail adequate to distinguish insidious chronic process from acute onset   [45] Yes_1 No_0 NA_9 XXXXXXXXXX

IF NO TO EITHER ITEM 4.a. OR b., chart should be subject to clinical review: [46] Appl_1 NA_9 XXXXXXXXXX

   Is assessment adequate?   XXXXXXXXXXXX   [47] Yes_1 No_0

   EXPLAIN:

5. Does patient have an SI score of less than 4 and a diagnosis of schizophrenia?   [48] Yes_1 No_0 XXXXXXXXXX

IF YES, chart should be subject to clinical review: [49] Appl_1 NA_9 XXXXXXXXXX

Was the diagnosis of this patient adequately established?	XXXXXXXXXXXX	^{50}Yes$_1$ No$_0$

6. Does patient have an SI score of 4 or more and a diagnosis other than schizophrenia? ^{74}Yes$_1$ No$_0$ NA$_9$ XXXXXXXXXX XXXXXXXXXX XXXXXXXXXX

IF YES, chart should be subject to clinical review: ^{75}Appl$_1$ NA$_9$ XXXXXXXXXX

Was the alternative diagnosis adequately established?   XXXXXXXXXXXX ^{76}Yes$_1$ No$_0$
EXPLAIN:

SCHIZOPHRENIC INDEX

Symptoms	PIAS Review	Points to be scored for YES response
1. *Delusions and hallucinations*		
a. Delusions (not specified or other than depressive?)	^{51}Yes$_1$ No$_0$	2
b. Hallucinations (auditory)	^{52}Yes$_1$ No$_0$	2
c. Hallucinations (visual)	^{53}Yes$_1$ No$_0$	(for any or all of
d. Hallucinations (other)	^{54}Yes$_1$ No$_0$	b, c, d)
2. *Crazy thinking and/or thought disorder*		
a. Bizarre thinking	^{55}Yes$_1$ No$_0$	2
b. Autism or grossly unrealistic private thoughts	^{56}Yes$_1$ No$_0$	(for any or all of a, b, c)
c. Looseness of association, illogical thinking, overinclusion	^{57}Yes$_1$ No$_0$	
d. Blocking	^{58}Yes$_1$ No$_0$	1 (for either or
e. Concreteness	^{59}Yes$_1$ No$_0$	both d, e)
f. Derealization	^{60}Yes$_1$ No$_0$	1
g. Depersonalization	^{61}Yes$_1$ No$_0$	1
3. *Inappropriate affect*	^{62}Yes$_1$ No$_0$	1
4. *Confusion*	^{63}Yes$_1$ No$_0$	1
5. *Paranoid ideation* (self-referential thinking, suspiciousness)	^{64}Yes$_1$ No$_0$	1
6. *Catatonic motor behavior*		
a. Excitement	^{65}Yes$_1$ No$_0$	1
b. Stupor	^{66}Yes$_1$ No$_0$	(for any or all of
c. Waxy flexibility	^{67}Yes$_1$ No$_0$	a. through g.)

d. Negativism ^{68}Yes$_1$ No$_0$
e. Mutism ^{69}Yes$_1$ No$_0$
f. Echolalia ^{70}Yes$_1$ No$_0$
g. Stereotyped motor activity ^{71}Yes$_1$ No$_0$

$^{72-73}$SCORE: _____ *

*Where the score would be less than 4 without inclusion of 2.d. and/or 2.e., these symptoms are not scored.

1. B.M. Astrachan, D. Adler, L. Brauer, M. Harrow, A. Schwartz, C. Schwartz, and G. Tucker, "A Checklist for the Diagnosis of Schizophrenia," working manuscript, Yale University, Department of Psychiatry, 1971.

G. *Medical Evaluation* XXXXXXXXXX
  1. Were any of the following indi- XXXXXXXXXX
    cated as present in the chart: XXXXXXXXXX
    a. Physical health rated poor or XXXXXXXXXX
      very poor on MSER or PER-C ^{8}Yes$_1$ No$_0$ XXXXXXXXXX
    b. Appetite rated poor or very XXXXXXXXXX
      poor on MSER or PER-C ^{9}Yes$_1$ No$_0$ XXXXXXXXXX
    c. Insomnia rated moderate or XXXXXXXXXX
      marked on MSER or PER-C ^{10}Yes$_1$ No$_0$ XXXXXXXXXX
    d. Unwarranted concern with XXXXXXXXXX
      physical health rated moderate XXXXXXXXXX
      or marked on MSER or PER-C ^{11}Yes$_1$ No$_0$ XXXXXXXXXX
    e. Severe sensory impairment XXXXXXXXXX
      (visual or hearing) (MSER or XXXXXXXXXX
      PER-C) ^{12}Yes$_1$ No$_0$ XXXXXXXXXX
    f. Patient acutely intoxicated on XXXXXXXXXX
      drugs or alcohol at time of XXXXXXXXXX
      evaluation ^{13}Yes$_1$ No$_0$ XXXXXXXXXX
    g. Suicidal patient with current XXXXXXXXXX
      injury ^{14}Yes$_1$ No$_0$ XXXXXXXXXX
    h. Diagnosis of schizophrenia XXXXXXXXXX
      (APA 295.0–295.99) ^{15}Yes$_1$ No$_0$ XXXXXXXXXX
    i. Diagnosis of organic brain syn- XXXXXXXXXX
      drome (APA 290.0–294.0 and XXXXXXXXXX
      309.0) ^{16}Yes$_1$ No$_0$ XXXXXXXXXX
    j. Patient is under 18 or over 45 ^{17}Yes$_1$ No$_0$ XXXXXXXXXX

    IF NO TO ALL ITEMS 1.a.–j., XXXXXXXXXX
    MARK NA IN CLINICAL XXXXXXXXXX
    REVIEW SECTION ITEM G.2 XXXXXXXXXX
    AND SKIP TO ITEM G.3 BELOW. XXXXXXXXXX

  2. IF YES to any item 1.a.–j., is there XXXXXXXXXX
    an indication in the chart of the XXXXXXXXXX
    following: XXXXXXXXXX
    a. Name of the patient's family XXXXXXXXXX
      physician or an indication that XXXXXXXXXX
      there is none ^{18}Yes$_1$ No$_0$ XXXXXXXXXX
    b. Approximate date (year) of XXXXXXXXXX
      the most recent physical check- XXXXXXXXXX
      up ^{19}Yes$_1$ No$_0$ XXXXXXXXXX
    c. Inquiry into past XXXXXXXXXX
      1) illnesses ^{20}Yes$_1$ No$_0$ XXXXXXXXXX
      2) operations ^{21}Yes$_1$ No$_0$ XXXXXXXXXX
      3) accidents ^{22}Yes$_1$ No$_0$ XXXXXXXXXX

d. Inquiry into family history of
   1) epilepsy   [23]Yes_1 No_0 XXXXXXXXXX
   2) suicide   [24]Yes_1 No_0 XXXXXXXXXX
   3) chronic or periodic mental   XXXXXXXXXX
       illness   [25]Yes_1 No_0 XXXXXXXXXX

IF NO to any item 2.a.–d., chart   XXXXXXXXXX
should be subject to clinical review: [26]Appl_1 NA_9 XXXXXXXXXX

Was the medical evaluation of
this patient sufficiently com-
plete and adequate?   XXXXXXXXXXXX   [27]Yes_1 No_0
EXPLAIN:

3. Did the chart indicate history or   XXXXXXXXXX
    presence of any of the following: XXXXXXXXXX
    a. faintings   [28]Yes_1 No_0 XXXXXXXXXX
    b. periodic headaches   [29]Yes_1 No_0 XXXXXXXXXX
    c. dizziness attacks   [30]Yes_1 No_0 XXXXXXXXXX
    d. seizures or spells   [31]Yes_1 No_0 XXXXXXXXXX
    e. head trauma   [32]Yes_1 No_0 XXXXXXXXXX
    f. impairment of consciousness,   XXXXXXXXXX
       orientation, or cognitive func-   XXXXXXXXXX
       tioning (See MSER or PER-C)   [33]Yes_1 No_0 XXXXXXXXXX
    g. fugue states   [34]Yes_1 No_0 XXXXXXXXXX

IF NO TO ALL ITEMS 3.a.–g.,   XXXXXXXXXX
MARK NA IN CLINICAL   XXXXXXXXXX
REVIEW SECTION, AND SKIP   XXXXXXXXXX
TO ITEM 4 BELOW.   XXXXXXXXXX

IF YES TO ANY ITEM 3.a.–g.,   XXXXXXXXXX
was a neurological examination or   XXXXXXXXXX
an examination by a neurological   XXXXXXXXXX
consultant performed?   [35]Yes_1 No_0 XXXXXXXXXX

IF NO, the chart should be sub-
ject to clinical review: [36]Appl_1 NA_9 XXXXXXXXXX

Was the medical evaluation of
this patient sufficiently com-
plete and adequate?   XXXXXXXXXXXX   [37]Yes_1 No_0
EXPLAIN:

4. Is patient pregnant?   [38]Yes_1 No_0 XXXXXXXXXX

IF NO, SKIP TO ITEM 5 BELOW.   XXXXXXXXXX

IF YES, does the chart indicate   XXXXXXXXXX
the following: XXXXXXXXXX
a. whether she is under the care   XXXXXXXXXX
    of an obstetrician and, if so,   XXXXXXXXXX
    his name   [39]Yes_1 No_0 XXXXXXXXXX

b. if medication was prescribed,
   was the obstetrician contacted ^{40}Yes$_1$ No$_0$ NA$_9$ XXXXXXXXXX
   XXXXXXXXXX
5. Is patient adolescent (over 12 and
   under 18) ^{41}Yes$_1$ No$_0$ XXXXXXXXXX
   XXXXXXXXXX

IF NO, MARK NA IN CLINICAL
REVIEW SECTION AND SKIP
TO SECTION H

XXXXXXXXXX
XXXXXXXXXX
XXXXXXXXXX

IF YES, does the chart indicate
any of the following:
   a. impulsive behavior ^{42}Yes$_1$ No$_0$
   b. spotty school record ^{43}Yes$_1$ No$_0$
   c. history of hyperkinetic
      childhood ^{44}Yes$_1$ No$_0$

XXXXXXXXXX
XXXXXXXXXX
XXXXXXXXXX
XXXXXXXXXX
XXXXXXXXXX
XXXXXXXXXX

IF NO TO ALL ITEMS 5.a.–c.,
MARK NA IN CLINICAL
REVIEW SECTION AND SKIP
TO SECTION H.

IF YES TO ANY ITEM 5.a.–c.,
was a detailed medical history
recorded? ^{45}Yes$_1$ No$_0$

XXXXXXXXXX
XXXXXXXXXX

    IF NO, chart should be subject
   to clinical review: ^{46}Appl$_1$ NA$_9$

XXXXXXXXXX
XXXXXXXXXX

       Was the medical evaluation
      adequate? XXXXXXXXXXXX ^{47}Yes$_1$ No$_0$
      EXPLAIN:

H. *Assessment for Suicide* XXXXXXXXXX
   1. Does the chart indicate that the XXXXXXXXXX
      suicidal potential of the patient XXXXXXXXXX
      was addressed? ^{48}Yes$_1$ No$_0$ XXXXXXXXXX
   2. IF YES, was patient considered XXXXXXXXXX
      as having not significant or low XXXXXXXXXX
      potential for suicide? ^{49}Yes$_1$ No$_0$ NA$_9$ XXXXXXXXXX

IF YES TO BOTH ITEMS 1 and 2,
MARK NA IN CLINICAL REVIEW
SECTIONS, ITEMS H.3–4, AND
SKIP TO SECTION I BELOW.

   3. IF NO TO EITHER ITEM 1 or 2, XXXXXXXXXX
      does the chart indicate that the XXXXXXXXXX
      following have been addressed: XXXXXXXXXX
      a. details of suicidal thoughts, XXXXXXXXXX
         gestures or attempts ^{50}Yes$_1$ No$_0$ XXXXXXXXXX
      b. individual or family history of XXXXXXXXXX
         prior suicidal behavior ^{51}Yes$_1$ No$_0$ XXXXXXXXXX
      c. assessment of current symp- XXXXXXXXXX
         toms such as depression, hos- XXXXXXXXXX
         tility, low impulse control, XXXXXXXXXX
         alcoholism, drug abuse or over- XXXXXXXXXX
         whelming anxiety of psychotic XXXXXXXXXX
         proportions ^{52}Yes$_1$ No$_0$ XXXXXXXXXX

    d. history of recent stresses,
including severe and acute
situational crises such as family
discord, loss of environmental
or social support, death of
significant person, threats to
personal freedom (i.e. draft) ^{53}Yes$_1$ No$_0$

XXXXXXXXXX
XXXXXXXXXX
XXXXXXXXXX
XXXXXXXXXX
XXXXXXXXXX
XXXXXXXXXX
XXXXXXXXXX

    e. history relevant to medical
status, such as chronic, serious
or incurable medical illness ^{54}Yes$_1$ No$_0$

XXXXXXXXXX
XXXXXXXXXX
XXXXXXXXXX

    f. social circumstances and
resources, such as financial,
availability of family and
friends, their reaction, whether
it is rejecting, unconcerned or
supportive, degree of social
isolation ^{55}Yes$_1$ No$_0$

XXXXXXXXXX
XXXXXXXXXX
XXXXXXXXXX
XXXXXXXXXX
XXXXXXXXXX
XXXXXXXXXX
XXXXXXXXXX

    g. attention to the communicative
aspects of the suicidal behavior,
what their goals are and
whether these goals are being
met ^{56}Yes$_1$ No$_0$

XXXXXXXXXX
XXXXXXXXXX
XXXXXXXXXX
XXXXXXXXXX
XXXXXXXXXX

IF NO to any item 2.a.–g.,
chart should be subject to
clinical review: ^{57}Appl$_1$ NA$_9$ XXXXXXXXXX

      Was the assessment for
suicide adequate?   XXXXXXXXXXXX ^{58}Yes$_1$ No$_0$
EXPLAIN:

4. If the chart indicates the presence
of any suicidal thoughts, gestures
or attempts, was the patient
offered treatment (in-patient or
out-patient)? ^{59}Yes$_1$ No$_0$ NA$_9$

XXXXXXXXXX
XXXXXXXXXX
XXXXXXXXXX
XXXXXXXXXX
XXXXXXXXXX

IF NO, chart should be subject to
clinical review: ^{60}Appl$_1$ NA$_9$ XXXXXXXXXX

      Was disposition appropriate?   XXXXXXXXXXXX ^{61}Yes$_1$ No$_0$
EXPLAIN:

I. *Assessment of Support*
    1. Does the chart indicate that the
patient has any of the following
characteristics:
      a. a diagnosis of psychotic dis-
order (APA 290–299) ^{53}Yes$_1$ No$_0$

XXXXXXXXXX
XXXXXXXXXX
XXXXXXXXXX
XXXXXXXXXX
XXXXXXXXXX
XXXXXXXXXX

   b. patient is in financial crisis
      being unable to support self
      or family ^{54}Yes$_1$ No$_0$
   c. social isolate ^{55}Yes$_1$ No$_0$
   d. an unemancipated minor ^{56}Yes$_1$ No$_0$
   e. over 65 years of age ^{57}Yes$_1$ No$_0$
   f. receiving aid from Welfare *or*
      income under $50 a week Yes$_1$ No$_0$

IF NO TO ALL ITEMS 1.a.–e.,
MARK NA IN CLINICAL REVIEW
SECTION, ITEM 2, AND SKIP TO
SECTION J BELOW.

2. IF YES TO ANY ITEM 1.a.–e.,
   have the following been addressed
   in the patient's record:
   a. degree of patient stress and
      distress ^{58}Yes$_1$ No$_0$
   b. strength of internal resources
      (reality testing, impulse con-
      trol, motivation, etc.). ^{59}Yes$_1$ No$_0$
   c. household composition ^{60}Yes$_1$ No$_0$
   d. interpersonal help available
      (family, friends, job, etc.) ^{61}Yes$_1$ No$_0$

IF NO TO ANY ITEM 2.a.–d.,
chart should be subject to clinical
review: ^{62}Appl$_1$ NA$_9$

Was assessment of support
adequate? ^{63}Yes$_1$ No$_0$
EXPLAIN:

J. *Formulation, Treatment Plan, Disposition*
  1. Are the following present in the
     chart:
    a. Formulation of problem (not
       necessarily a psychodynamic
       explanation of patient's
       development) ^{64}Yes$_1$ No$_0$
    b. Treatment plan, including one
       or more of the following:
       1) interventions needed
       2) types of treatment (group,
          family, inpatient, etc.)
       3) medication
       4) referral or discharge with-
          out treatment ^{65}Yes$_1$ No$_0$
    c. if patient was accepted for
       treatment at CMHC, was there
       an assessment of his motiva-
       tion, including degree of dis-

comfort, insight, resources he
is willing to commit to treat-
ment ^{66}Yes$_1$ No$_0$ NA$_9$

XXXXXXXXXX
XXXXXXXXXX
XXXXXXXXXX

IF NO TO ANY ITEM 1.a.–c.,
chart should be subject to clinical
review: ^{67}Appl$_1$ NA$_9$ XXXXXXXXXX

Was the formulation of the
patient's problem adequate for
the reviewer to assess the
treatment plan?   XXXXXXXXXXXX ^{68}Yes$_1$ No$_0$
EXPLAIN:

Was the treatment plan
recorded sufficiently well to
be independently assessed
by a reviewer?   XXXXXXXXXXXX ^{69}Yes$_1$ No$_0$
EXPLAIN:

Do you agree with the treat-
ment plan?   XXXXXXXXXXXX ^{70}Yes$_1$ No$_0$
EXPLAIN:

2. Is the disposition at intake present
   in the chart? ^{71}Yes$_1$ No$_0$ XXXXXXXXXX

IF YES, does the disposition
implement the treatment plan? ^{72}Yes$_1$ No$_0$ NA$_9$

IF NO TO EITHER QUESTION
ITEM 2, chart should be subject
to clinical review: ^{73}Appl$_1$ NA$_9$ XXXXXXXXXX

Was the disposition appropriate? XXXXXXXXXXXX ^{74}Yes$_1$ No$_0$
EXPLAIN:

3. Did the patient drop-out prior to
   mutually agreed upon treatment/
   referral/termination? ^{75}Yes$_1$ No$_0$ XXXXXXXXXX

Or, did patient sign out *against
medical advice?*

IF YES, chart should be subject
to clinical review: ^{76}Appl$_1$ NA$_9$ XXXXXXXXXX

Was the intake process appropriately and adequately
handled to prevent drop-out?   XXXXXXXXXXXX ^{77}Yes$_1$ No$_0$
EXPLAIN:

III.   *Adequacy of Treatment*   XXXXXXXXXX
A. *General*   XXXXXXXXXX
    1. Does the chart indicate patient⁻   XXXXXXXXXX
       was: XXXXXXXXXX
       a. actually admitted to treatment   XXXXXXXXXX
           in the CMHC? ^{8}Yes$_1$ No$_0$ XXXXXXXXXX
       b. given psychotropic medication   XXXXXXXXXX
           during the process of evalua-   XXXXXXXXXX
           tion? ^{9}Yes$_1$ No$_0$ XXXXXXXXXX
       c. over 12 and under 18? ^{10}Yes$_1$ No$_0$ XXXXXXXXXX
       d. rated as having a moderate to   XXXXXXXXXX
           very high degree of suicidal   XXXXXXXXXX
           potential? ^{11}Yes$_1$ No$_0$ XXXXXXXXXX

       IF NO TO ALL ITEMS 1.a.–d.,   XXXXXXXXXX
       TERMINATE REVIEW HERE   XXXXXXXXXX
       AND NOTE TIME REQUIRED   XXXXXXXXXX
       TO COMPLETE REVIEW ON   XXXXXXXXXX
       p. 274.   XXXXXXXXXX

    2. IF YES TO ITEM 1.a., did the   XXXXXXXXXX
       actual treatment provided follow   XXXXXXXXXX
       the treatment plan formulated at   XXXXXXXXXX
       intake? ^{12}Yes$_1$ No$_0$ XXXXXXXXXX

       IF NO, were the changes in plan   XXXXXXXXXX
       explained in the chart on the   XXXXXXXXXX
       basis of subsequent information   XXXXXXXXXX
       or events? ^{13}Yes$_1$ No$_0$ NA$_9$ XXXXXXXXXX

       IF NO, chart should be subject to
       clinical review: ^{14}Appl$_1$ NA$_9$ XXXXXXXXXX

           Do you agree with the changes
           in treatment plan?   XXXXXXXXXXXX ^{15}Yes$_1$ No$_0$
           EXPLAIN:

       IF YES to 1.b., complete section
         B. *Medication*.
       IF YES to 1.d., complete section
         C. *Treatment of Suicidal Patients*.
       IF YES to 1.c., complete section
         D. *Treatment of Adolescents*.

B. *Medication*   XXXXXXXXXX
    1. Is the chart clear about whether   XXXXXXXXXX
       or not medication was prescribed? ^{16}Yes$_1$ No$_0$ XXXXXXXXXX

2. IF YES, was medication prescribed? ^{17}Yes$_1$ No$_0$ XXXXXXXXXX
XXXXXXXXXX

IF NO TO EITHER ITEM 1 OR 2, XXXXXXXXXX
MARK NA IN CLINICAL REVIEW XXXXXXXXXX
SECTIONS, ITEMS 4. a.–c., 5 XXXXXXXXXX
AND 6, AND SKIP TO SECTION XXXXXXXXXX
C, p. 265. ^{18}Yes$_1$ No$_0$ XXXXXXXXXX

3. IF YES, does the chart indicate XXXXXXXXXX
the following: XXXXXXXXXX
   a. names of medication(s) ^{19}Yes$_1$ No$_0$ XXXXXXXXXX
   b. dosages ^{20}Yes$_1$ No$_0$ XXXXXXXXXX
   c. side effects or absence of side XXXXXXXXXX
      effects (NA if patient did not XXXXXXXXXX
      return) ^{21}Yes$_1$ No$_0$ NA$_9$ XXXXXXXXXX
   d. efficacy (NA if patient did not XXXXXXXXXX
      return) ^{22}Yes$_1$ No$_0$ NA$_9$ XXXXXXXXXX

IF NO TO EITHER ITEM 3.a XXXXXXXXXX
OR b., MARK NA IN CLINICAL XXXXXXXXXX
REVIEW SECTIONS, ITEMS 4. XXXXXXXXXX
a.–c., 5 AND 6 AND SKIP TO XXXXXXXXXX
SECTION C, p. 265. XXXXXXXXXX

4. If medication was prescribed and XXXXXXXXXX
adequately recorded, was it: XXXXXXXXXX
   a. a minor tranquilizer only ^{19}Yes$_1$ No$_0$ XXXXXXXXXX

   IF NO, MARK NA IN CLINI- XXXXXXXXXX
   CAL REVIEW SECTION AND XXXXXXXXXX
   SKIP TO ITEM 4.b. XXXXXXXXXX
   IF YES, was one or more of XXXXXXXXXX
   the following diagnostic num- XXXXXXXXXX
   bers given to the patient: 291, XXXXXXXXXX
   300–307, 309.13, 316? ^{20}Yes$_1$ No$_0$ XXXXXXXXXX

   IF NO, chart should be
   subject to clinical review: ^{21}Appl$_1$ NA$_9$ XXXXXXXXXX
   Was the medication
   adequate? XXXXXXXXXXXX ^{22}Yes$_1$ No$_0$
   EXPLAIN:

   Do you agree with the
   diagnosis given to this
   patient? XXXXXXXXXXXX ^{23}Yes$_1$ No$_1$
   EXPLAIN:

   b. a major tranquilizer ^{24}Yes$_1$ No$_0$ XXXXXXXXXX
   IF NO, MARK NA IN CLINI- XXXXXXXXXX
   CAL REVIEW SECTION AND XXXXXXXXXX
   SKIP TO ITEM 4.c. XXXXXXXXXX

was deferred in the interests of
developing a therapeutic alliance
with the adolescent? ^{65}Yes$_1$ No$_0$ NA$_9$ XXXXXXXXXX
XXXXXXXXXX
XXXXXXXXXX

IF NO, chart should be sub-
ject to clinical review: ^{66}Appl$_1$ NA$_9$ XXXXXXXXXX

Should parents have been
involved in evaluation or
treatment? XXXXXXXXXXXX ^{67}Yes$_1$ No$_0$
EXPLAIN:

4. Does the chart indicate any of
the following: XXXXXXXXXX
XXXXXXXXXX
   a. schizophrenic or other psy-
      chotic diagnosis (APA 295.0–
      299.0) ^{68}Yes$_1$ No$_0$ XXXXXXXXXX
XXXXXXXXXX
XXXXXXXXXX
   b. an idiosyncratic history (e.g.
      incest) ^{69}Yes$_1$ No$_0$ XXXXXXXXXX
XXXXXXXXXX
   c. anxiety rated moderate,
      marked or with episodes of
      panic (MSER or PER-C) ^{70}Yes$_1$ No$_0$ XXXXXXXXXX
XXXXXXXXXX
   d. state of ego disintegrity ^{71}Yes$_1$ No$_0$ XXXXXXXXXX

IF YES TO ANY OR ALL OF 4.a.–
d., was patient offered individual
treatment? ^{72}Yes$_1$ No$_0$ NA$_9$ XXXXXXXXXX
XXXXXXXXXX
XXXXXXXXXX

IF NO, chart should be subject
to clinical review: ^{73}Appl$_1$ NA$_9$ XXXXXXXXXX

Was the treatment of this
patient appropriate? XXXXXXXXXXXX ^{74}Yes$_1$ No$_0$
EXPLAIN:

5. Does the chart indicate: XXXXXXXXXX
XXXXXXXXXX
   a. a diagnosis of character dis-
      order (APA 301.0–301.9) ^{75}Yes$_1$ No$_0$ XXXXXXXXXX
   b. drug abuse ^{76}Yes$_1$ No$_0$ XXXXXXXXXX

IF YES TO EITHER a. OR b.,
was patient offered group treat-
ment? ^{77}Yes$_1$ No$_0$ NA$_9$ XXXXXXXXXX
XXXXXXXXXX
XXXXXXXXXX

IF NO TO PRECEDING ITEM,
chart should be subject to
clinical review: ^{8}Appl$_1$ NA$_9$ XXXXXXXXXX

Was the treatment of this
patient appropriate? XXXXXXXXXXXX ^{9}Yes$_1$ No$_0$
EXPLAIN:

6. If the patient was treated with group psychotherapy, was the group composed entirely of adolescents?

^{10}Yes$_1$ No$_0$ NA$_9$

XXXXXXXXXX
XXXXXXXXXX
XXXXXXXXXX
XXXXXXXXXX

IF NO, chart should be subject to clinical review:

^{11}Appl$_1$ NA$_9$ XXXXXXXXXX

Was the treatment of this patient appropriate? EXPLAIN:

XXXXXXXXXXXX ^{12}Yes$_1$ No$_0$

IV. *Review of Specific Treatment Services*
   A. *Inpatient Services*
      1. Does chart indicate:
         a. patient treated on an inpatient unit?

^{13}Yes$_1$ No$_0$

         b. suicidal potential rated moderate, high or very high?

^{14}Yes$_1$ No$_0$

XXXXXXXXXX
XXXXXXXXXX
XXXXXXXXXX
XXXXXXXXXX
XXXXXXXXXX
XXXXXXXXXX
XXXXXXXXXX

IF NO TO BOTH ITEMS 1.a. AND b., MARK NA IN CLINICAL REVIEW SECTION ITEM 2, AND SKIP TO SECTION B, p. 269.

XXXXXXXXXX
XXXXXXXXXX
XXXXXXXXXX
XXXXXXXXXX

IF YES TO EITHER 1.a. OR b., COMPLETE THE CRITERIA FOR HOSPITALIZATION CHECKLIST, BELOW AND RETURN TO ITEM 2.

XXXXXXXXXX
XXXXXXXXXX
XXXXXXXXXX
XXXXXXXXXX

2. Does patient have a criteria for hospitalization score of 11 or less and was given inpatient treatment at CMHC?

^{15}Yes$_1$ No$_0$

IF YES, chart should be subject to clinical review:

^{16}Appl$_1$ NA$_9$ XXXXXXXXXX

Was the treatment appropriate? EXPLAIN:

XXXXXXXXXXXX ^{17}Yes$_1$ No$_0$

PIAS Review Only

CRITERIA FOR HOSPITALIZATION[1]

Instructions to reviewers: 1) Rate patient on each criterion as: none = 0, slight = 1, moderate = 2, extensive = 3; multiply the ratio by the weight shown and enter the score on each criterion. Then sum scores on each criterion for total score. 2) Ratings are to be based on the patient's condition in the seven days preceding evaluation for hospitalization. 3) In applying the criteria, an item of reported behavior should be employed to arrive at a rating on the first criterion on the list to which it applies, *do not use* the *same* item of behavior to

1. This set of criteria constitutes a modification of the criteria proposed by H.G. Whittington, M.D., *Psychiatry in the American Community*, New York: International Universities Press, Inc., 1966.

score a criterion that falls later in the list (e.g. suicidal behavior should not be used in rating criteria numbers 4 and 5).

		Weight	*Score*
1.	Is there evidence of active suicidal preoccupation, in fantasy or thoughts of patient?	2	18
2.	Have there been suicidal attempts or active preparations to harm self (i.e. buying a gun, etc.)?	4	19–20
3.	Has the patient threatened to hurt someone else physically? (Limit to *verbal* threats)	2	21
4.	Have aggressive outbursts occurred toward people?	4	22
5.	Have aggressive outbursts occurred toward animals or objects?	2	23
6.	Has antisocial behavior occurred?	1	24
7.	Are there evidences of impairment of such functions as reality assessment, judgment, logical thinking, and planning?	1	25
8.	Does the patient's condition seem to be deteriorating rapidly or failing to improve despite supportive measures?	1	26
9.	Are there physical or neurological conditions *or* a psychotic, disorganized state which require(s) hospitalization to initiate the treatment process?	2	27
10.	Does a pathological or noxious situation exist among patient's family or associates that makes initiation of treatment without hospitalization impossible? *Or* does the patient's disordered state create such difficulties for family or associates that he has to be removed and hospitalized for their sake?	1	28
11.	Are emotional contacts of the patient so severely limited or the habitual patterns of behavior so pathologically ingrained that the "push" of a structured hospital program may be helpful? (This criterion should not be applied to acute patients, but only to those who are so limited as to be unable to establish and maintain emotional contacts.)	1	29
12.	Does evaluation of the patient's condition require the 24-hour observation and special evaluation that a hospital provides? (Including stabilization or re-evaluation of medication.) Or is patient referred for treatment of drug or alcohol dependence?	4	30–31
	TOTAL SCORE		32–33

B. *Outpatient Psychotherapy*

    1. Was patient treated in an individual or group outpatient psychotherapy unit? ^{34}Yes$_1$ No$_0$ XXXXXXXXXX XXXXXXXXXX XXXXXXXXXX XXXXXXXXXX

    IF NO, MARK NA IN CLINICAL REVIEW SECTION ITEM 2, AND SKIP TO SECTION C.   XXXXXXXXXX XXXXXXXXXX XXXXXXXXXX

    2. IF YES, which of the following defense mechanisms were identified: XXXXXXXXXX XXXXXXXXXX XXXXXXXXXX

      a. denial ^{35}Yes$_1$ No$_0$ XXXXXXXXXX

      b. repression ^{36}Yes$_1$ No$_0$ XXXXXXXXXX

      c. reaction formation ^{37}Yes$_1$ No$_0$ XXXXXXXXXX

d. sublimation	[38] Yes$_1$ No$_0$	XXXXXXXXXX
e. regression	[39] Yes$_1$ No$_0$	XXXXXXXXXX
f. projection	[40] Yes$_1$ No$_0$	XXXXXXXXXX
g. introjection	[41] Yes$_1$ No$_0$	XXXXXXXXXX
h. incorporation	[42] Yes$_1$ No$_0$	XXXXXXXXXX
i. identification	[43] Yes$_1$ No$_0$	XXXXXXXXXX
j. compartmentalization or		XXXXXXXXXX
isolation	[44] Yes$_1$ No$_0$	XXXXXXXXXX
k. conversion	[45] Yes$_1$ No$_0$	XXXXXXXXXX
l. displacement	[46] Yes$_1$ No$_0$	XXXXXXXXXX
m. compensation	[47] Yes$_1$ No$_0$	XXXXXXXXXX
n. undoing	[48] Yes$_1$ No$_0$	XXXXXXXXXX
o. somatization	[49] Yes$_1$ No$_0$	XXXXXXXXXX
p. symbolization	[50] Yes$_1$ No$_0$	XXXXXXXXXX
q. rationalization	Yes No	XXXXXXXXXX

IF NO TO ALL ITEMS 2.a.–p.,
chart should be subject to
clinical review: [51] Appl$_1$ NA$_9$ XXXXXXXXXX

Was the treatment (or
choice of treatment)
adequate? XXXXXXXXXXXX [52] Yes$_1$ No$_0$
EXPLAIN:

3. Were behavioral changes envisioned   XXXXXXXXXX
   for this patient? [53] Yes$_1$ No$_0$ XXXXXXXXXX

4. Does the chart indicate that the   XXXXXXXXXX
   length of contract (open-ended   XXXXXXXXXX
   more than three months) was dis-   XXXXXXXXXX
   cussed with the patient? [54] Yes$_1$ No$_0$ XXXXXXXXXX

C. *Outpatient Brief Treatment*   XXXXXXXXXX
   1. Was patient treated in an outpa-   XXXXXXXXXX
      tient brief treatment unit? [55] Yes$_1$ No$_0$ XXXXXXXXXX

IF NO, MARK NA IN CLINICAL   XXXXXXXXXX
REVIEW SECTION ITEM 2, AND   XXXXXXXXXX
SKIP TO SECTION D.   XXXXXXXXXX

2. IF YES,   XXXXXXXXXX
   a. Was the goal(s) of the present   XXXXXXXXXX
      contract defined? [56] Yes$_1$ No$_0$ XXXXXXXXXX
   b. Were the external precipitating   XXXXXXXXXX
      factors defined? [57] Yes$_1$ No$_0$ XXXXXXXXXX
   c. During the last year was the   XXXXXXXXXX
      patient at least six continuous   XXXXXXXXXX
      months without psychiatric   XXXXXXXXXX
      treatment? [58] Yes$_1$ No$_0$ XXXXXXXXXX
   d. If medication was given, were   XXXXXXXXXX
      the target symptoms defined? [59] Yes$_1$ No$_0$ NA$_9$ XXXXXXXXXX

IF NO TO ANY ITEM 2.a.–d.,
chart should be subject to clinical
review: [60] Appl$_1$ NA$_9$ XXXXXXXXXX

Was the treatment (or choice
of treatment) adequate?
EXPLAIN:
XXXXXXXXXXXX ^{61}Yes$_1$ No$_0$

3. Does the chart indicate that the
   length of the contract (no more
   than 12 weeks) was discussed
   with the patient? ^{62}Yes$_1$ No$_0$
XXXXXXXXXX
XXXXXXXXXX
XXXXXXXXXX
XXXXXXXXXX

D. *Continuing Care-Medication*
   Maintenance Program
   1. Was patient admitted to Continu-
      ing Care-Medication Maintenance
      Program? ^{63}Yes$_1$ No$_0$
XXXXXXXXXX
XXXXXXXXXX
XXXXXXXXXX
XXXXXXXXXX
XXXXXXXXXX

IF NO, MARK NA IN CLINICAL
REVIEW SECTION ITEMS 2 AND 3,
AND SKIP TO SECTION E.
XXXXXXXXXX
XXXXXXXXXX
XXXXXXXXXX

2. IF YES, does the chart indicate
   that the goals of treatment were:
   a. to prevent psychiatric hospital-
      ization and/or to prevent acute
      exacerbation of psychosis ^{64}Yes$_1$ No$_0$
   b. to help patient keep his job or
      other social activities with
      which he is involved ^{65}Yes$_1$ No$_0$
   c. to provide social contacts to
      counteract the isolation due to
      bad living conditions or other
      factors ^{66}Yes$_1$ No$_0$
   d. to rehabilitate patient through
      exposure to social interactions
      in a group activity, or occupa-
      tional therapy, or other forms
      of long-term treatment ^{67}Yes$_1$ No$_0$
XXXXXXXXXX
XXXXXXXXXX
XXXXXXXXXX
XXXXXXXXXX
XXXXXXXXXX
XXXXXXXXXX
XXXXXXXXXX
XXXXXXXXXX
XXXXXXXXXX
XXXXXXXXXX
XXXXXXXXXX
XXXXXXXXXX
XXXXXXXXXX
XXXXXXXXXX
XXXXXXXXXX
XXXXXXXXXX
XXXXXXXXXX

IF NO TO ALL ITEMS 2.a.–d.,
OR IF THE AIMS OF THE CON-
TRACT ARE NOT DEFINED,
chart should be subject to clinical
review: ^{68}Appl$_1$ NA$_9$ XXXXXXXXXX

Was the treatment adequate?
EXPLAIN:
XXXXXXXXXXXX ^{69}Yes$_1$ No$_0$

3. Is the name of the physician
   responsible for medical back-up
XXXXXXXXXX
XXXXXXXXXX

and supervision recorded in the
chart? ^{70}Yes$_1$ No$_0$ XXXXXXXXXX
XXXXXXXXXX

4. Does the patient attend the clinic
at least once a month or, if not, is
there a full rationale given for
other frequency of visits? ^{71}Yes$_1$ No$_0$ XXXXXXXXXX
XXXXXXXXXX
XXXXXXXXXX
XXXXXXXXXX

5. If the patient on medication missed
one or more appointments, does
the chart indicate that attempts
were made to contact him? (tele-
phone call, letter, home visit, etc.) ^{72}Yes$_1$ No$_0$ NA$_9$ XXXXXXXXXX
XXXXXXXXXX
XXXXXXXXXX
XXXXXXXXXX
XXXXXXXXXX

IF NO TO ANY ITEM 3–5, chart
should be subject to clinical review: ^{73}Appl$_1$ NA$_9$ XXXXXXXXXX

Was the treatment adequate? XXXXXXXXXXXX ^{74}Yes$_1$ No$_0$
EXPLAIN:

E. *Day Hospitalization Services* XXXXXXXXXX
1. Was patient admitted *directly* to a XXXXXXXXXX
day hospital unit? ^{8}Yes$_1$ No$_0$ XXXXXXXXXX

IF NO, MARK NA IN CLINICAL XXXXXXXXXX
REVIEW SECTION ITEM 2, AND XXXXXXXXXX
SKIP TO ITEM 3. XXXXXXXXXX

2. IF YES, XXXXXXXXXX
   a. Is there evidence presented XXXXXXXXXX
   that the patient was exposed to XXXXXXXXXX
   a current stressful (crisis) situa- XXXXXXXXXX
   tion that requires close collabo- XXXXXXXXXX
   ration of CMHC with any of XXXXXXXXXX
   the following: XXXXXXXXXX
   1) family ^{9}Yes$_1$ No$_0$ XXXXXXXXXX
   2) friends ^{10}Yes$_1$ No$_0$ XXXXXXXXXX
   3) employer ^{11}Yes$_1$ No$_0$ XXXXXXXXXX
   4) school ^{12}Yes$_1$ No$_0$ XXXXXXXXXX
   b. Does the record indicate that XXXXXXXXXX
   the patient was either psychotic XXXXXXXXXX
   or depressed (see diagnosis) XXXXXXXXXX
   and required immediate treat- XXXXXXXXXX
   ment with a high dosage of XXXXXXXXXX
   medication (see Treatment XXXXXXXXXX
   Plan)? ^{13}Yes$_1$ No$_0$ XXXXXXXXXX

IF YES: XXXXXXXXXX
   1) did the medical evaluation XXXXXXXXXX
   show him to be in good XXXXXXXXXX
   physical health? ^{14}Yes$_1$ No$_0$ NA$_9$ XXXXXXXXXX
   2) was the family able to pro- XXXXXXXXXX
   vide adequate support and XXXXXXXXXX
   ability to care for him XXXXXXXXXX
   evenings and weekends? ^{15}Yes$_1$ No$_0$ NA$_9$ XXXXXXXXXX

c. Does the record indicate that the patient required an intensive medical diagnostic work-up that could be more easily accomplished if patient were partially hospitalized? ^{16}Yes$_1$ No$_0$ XXXXXXXXXX XXXXXXXXXX XXXXXXXXXX XXXXXXXXXX XXXXXXXXXX XXXXXXXXXX

d. Does the record indicate that the patient required an intensive psychiatric diagnostic work-up that could be more easily accomplished if the patient were partially hospitalized? ^{17}Yes$_1$ No$_0$ XXXXXXXXXX XXXXXXXXXX XXXXXXXXXX XXXXXXXXXX XXXXXXXXXX XXXXXXXXXX

e. Does the record indicate that the patient's treatment program was oriented primarily towards outpatient therapy *but* that due to the patient's mental status (depression, psycho-motor retardation, lack of plans) the patient needed a structured program in order to "get going"? ^{18}Yes$_1$ No$_0$ XXXXXXXXXX XXXXXXXXXX XXXXXXXXXX XXXXXXXXXX XXXXXXXXXX XXXXXXXXXX XXXXXXXXXX XXXXXXXXXX XXXXXXXXXX

IF NO TO ALL ITEMS 2.a.–e., chart should be subject to clinical review: ^{19}Appl$_1$ NA$_9$ XXXXXXXXXX

Was partial hospitalization appropriate in this case?   XXXXXXXXXXXX ^{20}Yes$_1$ No$_0$
EXPLAIN:

3. Was patient *transferred* from 24-hour hospitalization to day hospital status? ^{21}Yes$_1$ No$_0$ XXXXXXXXXX XXXXXXXXXX XXXXXXXXXX

   IF NO, MARK NA IN CLINICAL REVIEW SECTION ITEM 4, AND TERMINATE REVIEW HERE XXXXXXXXXX XXXXXXXXXX XXXXXXXXXX

4. IF YES, does the record indicate that the patient improved during his initial 24-hour hospitalization but still needed to spend a significant amount of time in the hospital program for any of the following reasons:
   a. mental status ^{22}Yes$_1$ No$_0$
   b. nature of medication ^{23}Yes$_1$ No$_0$
   c. need for structured program ^{24}Yes$_1$ No$_0$
   d. completion of planning for discharge ^{25}Yes$_1$ No$_0$

   XXXXXXXXXX XXXXXXXXXX XXXXXXXXXX XXXXXXXXXX XXXXXXXXXX XXXXXXXXXX XXXXXXXXXX XXXXXXXXXX XXXXXXXXXX XXXXXXXXXX XXXXXXXXXX XXXXXXXXXX

IF NO TO ALL ITEMS 4.a.–d., chart should be subject to clinical review: ^{26}Appl$_1$ NA$_9$ XXXXXXXXXX

Was partial hospitalization
appropriate in this case?   XXXXXXXXXXXX ^{27}Yes$_1$ No$_0$
EXPLAIN:

Comments of Second Level Reviewer (e.g., inadequacies in chart not
covered in checklist):

TIME REQUIRED TO COMPLETE PIAS REVIEW: _____

References

Chapter one

1. Lee RL, Jones LW: The Fundamentals of Good Medical Care: An outline of the fundamentals of good medical care and an estimate of the service required to supply the medical needs of the United States. (*Publications of the Committee on the Costs of Medical Care No. 22*). (Chicago: University of Chicago Press, 1933).

2. Payne BC: Function of the audit committee in the general hospital. *Hospitals* 37:62–72, 1963.

3. Zusman J, Slawson MR: Service quality profile. *Arch Gen Psychiat* 27:692–698, 1972.

4. Plunkett RJ, Gordon JE: *Epidemiology and Mental Illness.* (New York: Basic Books, 1960).

5. Dohrenwend B, Dohrenwend B: *Social Status and Psychological Disorder: A Causal Inquiry.* (New York: John Wiley & Sons, 1969).

6. Beck AT, Ward CH, Mendelson M, Mack J, Erbaugh J. Reliability of psychiatric diagnoses. *Amer J Psychiat,* 119:351–357, 1962.

7. Babigian HM, Gardner EA, Miles HC, Romano J. Diagnostic consistency in a follow-up study of 1215 patients. *Amer J Psychiat,* 121:895–901, 1965.

8. Kendall RE, Cooper JE, Gourlay JRM, Copelan LS, Gurland BJ: Diagnostic criteria of American and British psychiatrists. *Arch Gen Psychiat,* 25:123–130, 1971.

9. Schmidt HO, Fonda CP: The reliability of psychiatric diagnosis: a new look. *J Abnorm Soc Psychol,* 52:262–267, 1956.

10. Silverman C. *The Epidemiology of Depression.* (Baltimore: *The Johns Hopkins Press,* 1968).

11. Ward CH, Beck AT, Mendelson M, Mock JE, Erbaugh J: The psychiatric nomenclature: reasons for diagnostic disagreement. *Arch Gen Psychiat,* 7: 198–205, 1962.

12. Luborsky L: Clinicians' judgments of mental health. *Arch Gen Psychiat,* 7:407–417, 1962.

13. Raskin A, Schulterbrandt J, Reatig N: Factors of psychopathology in interview, ward behavior and self-report ratings of hospitalized depressives. *J Consult Psychol,* 31: 270–278, 1967.
14. Hogarty GW, Ulrich G. The discharge readiness inventory. *Arch Gen Psychiat,* 25: 419–426, 1972.
15. Myers JK, Lindenthal JJ, Pepper MP: Life events and psychiatric impairment. *J. Nerv Ment Dis,* 152: 149–157, 1971.
16. Donabedian A: Evaluating the quality of medical care. *Milbank Mem Fund Quart, No. 2,* 44: 166–206, 1966.
17. Zusman J, Rieff ER: Evaluation of the quality of mental health services. *Arch Gen Psychiat,* 20:353–357, 1969.
18. Fox PD, Rappaport M: Some approaches to evaluating community mental health services. *Arch Gen Psychiat,* 26: 172–178, 1972.
19. Pugh TF, MacMahon B: Measurement of discontinuity of psychiatric inpatient care, *Public Health Reports,* 82:533–538, 1967.
20. McCaffreee KM: The cost of mental health care under changing treatment methods. *AJPH,* 56:1013–1025, 1966.
21. Ellsworth RB, Dickman HR, Maroney RJ: Characteristics of productive and unproductive unit systems in VA psychiatric hospitals. *Hosp Comm Psychiat,* 23:261–268, 1972.
22. Blackburn HL: Factors affecting turnover rates in mental hospitals. *Hosp Comm Psychiat,* 23:268–271, 1972.
23. Ullmann LP, Gurel L: Size, staffing and psychiatric hospital effectiveness: *Arch Gen Psychiat,* 11:360–367, 1964.
24. Tischler GL, Henisz J, Myers J, Garrison V. Catchmenting and the use of mental health services. *Arch Gen Psychiat,* 27:389–392, 1972.
25. Tischler GL, Henisz J, Myers J, Garrison V: The impact of catchmenting, *Administration in Mental Health,* 1:22–29, 1972.
26. Lembcke PA: Evaluation of the medical audit. *JAMA,* 199:111–118, 1967.
27. Morehead M: The medical audit as an operational tool. *Amer J Public Health,* 57:1643–1656, 1967.
28. Shindell S: *A Method of Hospital Utilization Review–HUP.* (Pittsburgh: University of Pittsburgh Press, 1966).
29. Kessner DM, Kalk CE, Singer J: Assessing health quality—the case for tracers. *New Eng J Med,* 288; 189–194, 1973.
30. Riedel DC, Fitzpatrick TB: *Patterns of Patient Care.* (Ann Arbor: University of Michigan Press, 1964).
31. Richman A, Pinsker H: Utilization review of psychiatric Inpatient care. *Amer J Psychiat* 130: 900–903, 1973.
32. Sheldon A: An evaluation of psychiatric after-care. *Br J Psychiatr,* 110: 662–667, 1964.
33. Pasamanick B, Scarpitti FR, Dinitz S: *Schizophrenics in the Community.* (New York: Appleton-Century-Crofts, 1967).

Chapter three

1. Pinel, Philippe, *A Treatise on Insanity,* trans. from the French ed., 1906 by D.D. Davis (New York: Hafner Publishing Company, 1962).

2. Meyer A, "The Collected Papers of Adolf Meyer," vol. 3, ed. by E.E. Winters, The Johns Hopkins Press, 1951.

3. Cheney CO, *Outlines for Psychiatric Examinations* (Utica: State Hospitals Press, 1934).

4. Donelly J, ed., *Outline of the Medical Record* (Hartford: Institute of Living, 1959).

5. Kirby GH: *Guides for History Taking and Clinical Examination of Psychiatric Cases,* Utica State Hospitals Press, 1921.

6. Lewis NDC: *Outlines for Psychiatric Examinations,* 3rd ed. (Utica: State Hospitals Press, 1934).

7. Preu PW: *Outline of Psychiatric Case Study* (New York: Paul B. Hoeber, Harper & Bros., 1933).

8. Beckett Peter, Grisell J, Crandall R and Gudobba R: "A Method of Formalizing Psychiatric Study," *Arch. Gen. Psychiat.* (Chicago) 16: 407–415, 1967.

9. Noyes AP, Kolb LC: *Modern Clinical Psychiatry,* ed. 6 (Philadelphia: W.B. Saunders Company, 1963).

10. Kerry RJ, Orme JE: "Psychiatric Diagnosis and the Inpatient Multidimensional Psychiatric Scale (I.M.P.S.)," *Br. J. Psychiat.* 121: 541–545, 1972.

11. Derogatis LR, Lipman RS, Covi L: "SCL–90: An Outpatient Psychiatric Rating Scale—Preliminary Report," *Psychopharmacol. Bull.* 9:13–28, 1973.

12. Denney Duane: "A Record Keeping System for a Psychiatric Consultation Service," *J. Nerv. Dis.* 141:474–477, 1966.

13. Ullmann LP, Alto P, Gurel, L: "Validity of Symptom Rating from Psychiatric Records," *Arch. Gen. Psychiat.* 7:130–134, 1962.

14. Jenkins RL, Stauffacher J, Hester R: "A Symptom Rating Scale for Use with Psychotic Patients," *Arch. Gen. Psychiat.* 1:197–204, 1959.

15. Shaffer JW, Nussbaum K, Lewis SM: "Psychiatric Assessment from Documentary Evidence," *Compr. Psychiat.* 12:564–571, 1971.

16. Weed LL: "Medical Records that Guide and Teach," *New England J. Med.* 278:593–600, 652–657, 1968.

17. Weed LL: *Medical Records, Medical Education and Patient Care* (Cleveland: Case Western Reserve University, 1969).

18. Bjorn JC, Cross HD: *The Problem-Oriented Private Practice of Medicine.* (New York: McGraw Hill, 1970).

19. Grant RL, Maletzky BM: "A Scientific Approach to Psychiatric Record Keeping," *Psychiat. Med.* 3:119–129, 1972.

20. Hayes-Roth R, Longabaugh R, Ryback R: "The Problem-Oriented Medical Record and Psychiatry," *Br. J. Psychiat.* 121:27–34, 1972.

21. Ryback Ralph S, Gardner JS: "Problem Formulation: The Problem-Oriented Record," *Amer. J. Psychiat.* 130:132–316, 1973.

22. Novello Joseph R: "The Problem-Oriented Record in Psychiatry," *J. Nerv. Ment. Dis.* 156:349–353, 1973.

23. Donnelly John, Rosenberg M, Fleeson W: "The Evolution of the Mental Status Past and Future," *Amer. J. Psychiat.* 126:997-1002, 1970.
24. Endicott Jean, Spitzer RL: "Current and Past Psychopathology Scales (CAPPS) Rationale, Reliability, and Validity," *Arch. Gen. Psychiat.* 27:678-687, 1972.
25. Lorr Maurice, Hamlin RM: "Estimation of the Major Psychotic Disorders by Objective Test Scores," *J. Nerv. Ment. Dis.* 151:219-224, 1970.
26. Lorr Maurice, Hamlin RM: "A Multimethod Factor Analysis of Behavioral and Objective Measures of Psychopathology," *J. Consult. Clin. Psychol.* 36:136-141, 1971.
27. Nathan Zare, Simpton S, Harriet F, Andberg M: "A System Analytic Model of Diagnosis: I. The Diagnostic Validity of Abnormal Psychomotor Behavior," *J. Clin. Psychology* 25:3-9, 1969.
28. Fleiss Joseph, Gurland BJ, Cooper JE: "Some Contributions to the Measurement of Psychopathology," *Br. J. Psychiat.* 119:647-656, 1971.
29. Spitzer RL, Fleiss JL, Endicott J, Cohen J: "Mental Status Schedule: Properties of Factor-Analytically Derived Scales," *Arch. Gen. Psychiat.* 16:479-493, 1967.
30. Spitzer RL, Endicott J, Fleiss JL, Cohen J: "The Psychiatric Status Schedule. A Technique for Evaluating and Psychopathology and Impairment in Role Functioning," *Arch. Gen. Psychiat.* 23:41-55, 1970.
31. Endicott J, Spitzer RL: "What! Another Rating Scale? The Psychiatric Evaluation Form," *J. Nerv. Ment. Dis.* 154:88-104, 1972.
32. Lorr M, Klett, CJ: *Inpatient Multidimensional Psychiatric Scale.* (Palo Alto, California: Consulting Psychologists Press, 1967).
33. Lorr M, Klett CJ: "Major Psychotic Disorders," *Arch. Gen. Psychiat.* 19:652-658, 1966.
34. Lorr M, Klett CJ: "Cross-cultural Comparison of Psychotic Syndromes," *J. Abnormal Psychology* 74:531-543, 1969.
35. Lorr M, Klett CJ: "Psychotic Behavioural Types," *Arch. Gen. Psychiat.* 20:592-597, 1969b.
36. Laska Eugene, Morrill D, Kline SS, Hackett E, Simpson, GM: "SCRIBE— A Method for Producing Automated Narrative Psychiatric, Case Histories," *Amer. J. Psychiat.* 124:82-84, 1967.
37. Glueck Bernad S: "The Use of Computers in Patient Care," *J. Hospital and Community Psychiatry* 16:117-120, 1965.
38. Richman A: "Computer Processing of Routine Psychiatric Records," *Meth. Inform. Med.* 5:25-30, 1966.
39. Eiduson Bernice, Brooks SH, Motto RL: "A Generalized Psychiatric Information-Processing System," *Behavioral Science* 11:133-142, 1966.
40. Ledley RS, Lusted LB: "The Use of Electronic Computers in Medical Data Processing: Aids in Diagnosis, Current Information Retrieval,

and Medical Record Keeping," *IRE Transactions Biomed. Trans. ME* 7:31–47, 1960.

41. Brenner M. Harvey, Paris H: "Records Systems for Hospital Outpatient Clinics," Supplement to *Medical Care,* 11:41–50, 1973.
42. Smith Alwyn, Birm DPH: "Automation of Medical Record-Keeping," *Lancet* 1:395–397, 1964.
43. Goldstein DH: "The Use of Medical Records to Yield Maximum Information: Methods for Different-Sized Plants—A Symposium," *J. Occupational Medicine* 5:128–144, 1963.
44. Goldstein DH, Benvit JN: "The Experience of a Medium-Sized Company," *J. Occupational Medicine* 5:128–144, 1963.
45. Palmer HH, Heyburn MC: "Methods Applicable to a Small Plant," *J. Occupational Medicine* 5:128–144, 1963.
46. Pell S: "The Experience of a Large Company," *J. Occupational Medicine* 5:128–144, 1963.
47. Baldwin JA: "Aspects of the Epidemiology of Mental Illness: Studies in Record Linkage, Preface, *Int. Psychiat. Clin.* 7(4): VII–XII, 1971.
48. Gorwitz Kurt, Bahn AK, Chandler CA, Martin WA: "Planned Uses of a Statewide Psychiatric Register for Aiding Mental Health in the Community," *Amer. J. Orthopsychiat.* 33:494–500, 1963.
49. Gardner EA: "The Use of a Psychiatric Case Register in the Planning and Evaluation of a Mental Health Program," Psychiat. Research *Reports of the American Psychiatric Association* 22:259–281, 1967.
50. Bahn AK: "A Psychiatric Case Register Conference," *Amer. J. Psychiat.* 119:878–879, 1963.
51. Laska E, Simpson GM, Bank R: "A Computerized Mental Status," *Compr. Psychiat.* 10:135–146, 1969.
52. Sletten WI, Ernhart CB, Ulett GA: "The Missouri Automated Mental Status Examination: Development, Use and Reliability," *Compr. Psychiat.* 11:315–327, 1970.
53. Benfari RC, Leighton AH, Beiser M, Coen K: "Case: Computer Assigned Symptom Evaluation. An Instrument for Psychiatric Epidemiological Application," *J. Nerv. Ment. Dis.* 154:115–125, 1972.
54. Graham JR: "Feedback and Accuracy of Predications of Hospitalization from the MMPI," *J. Clin. Psycholo.* 27:243–245, 1971.

Chapter four

1. Blum RH: Case Identification in Psychiatric Epidemiology. Methods and Problems. *The Milbank Memorial Fund Quart.* 3:253–288, 1962.
2. Gurin G, Veroff J, Feld S. *Americans View Their Mental Health: A Nationwide Survey.* (New York: Basic Books, 1960).
3. Katz MM, Lyerly SB. Methods for Measuring Adjustment and Social Behavior in the Community. *Psychol Reports* 13:503–535, 1963.
4. McMillan AM: The Health Opinion Survey: Technique for Estimating Prevalence of Psychoneurotic and Related Disorders in Communities. *Psychological Reports* 3:325–339, 1957.

5. Manis JG, Brawer MJ, Hunt CL, Kercher LC. Validating a Mental Health Scale. *Amer Sociol Rev* 29:84–89, 1964.
6. Phillips DL. The "True Prevalence" of Mental Illness in a New England State. *Community Mental Health J.* 2:35–40, 1966.
7. Richman A. Assessing the Need for Psychiatric Care; a Review of Validity of Psychiatric Surveys. *Can Psychiat Assn J.* 11:179–188, 1966.
8. Schwartz CC, Myers JK, Astrachan BM. Comparing Three Measures of Mental Status: A Note on the Validity of Estimates of Psychological Disorder in the Community. *J Health Soc Behav* 14:265–273, 1973.
9. Spiro HR, Siassi I, Crocetti G. What Gets Surveyed in a Psychiatric Survey? In Case Study of the MacMillan Index. *J. Nerv Ment Dis* 152:105–114, 1972.
10. Srole L, Langner TS, Michael ST, Opler MK, Rennie TAC. Mental Health in the Metropolis: *The Midtown Manhattan Study,* Vol 1. (New York: McGraw Hill, 1962).
11. Cochran DG. Methodological Problems in the Study of Human Population. *Ann. N.Y. Academy of Sciences,* 107:476–489, 1963.
12. Redick RW, Goldsmith HF. 1970 Census Data Used to Indicate Areas with Different Potentials for Mental Health and Related Problems. *Methodology Reports,* Mental Health Statistics, Series C, No. 3, DHEW Publications No. (HSM) 73–9058, 1972.
13. Rosen BM. A Model for Estimating Mental Health Needs Using 1970 Census Socioeconomic Data. *Methodology Reports,* Mental Health Statistics Series C, No. 9, DHEW Publication No. (ADM) 74–63, 1974.
14. Dohrenwend BP, Dohrenwend BS. *Social Status and Psychological Disorder: A Causal Inquiry.* (New York: John Wiley & Sons, 1969).
15. Haberman DW. An Analysis of Retest Scores for an Index of Psychophysiological Disturbance. *J Health & Human Behavior* 6:257–260, 1965.
16. Tyhurst JS. The Role of Transition States—Including Disasters—in Mental Illness. *Symposium on Preventive and Social Psychiatry,* Washington, DC, *Govt Printing Office* 149–69, 1957.
17. Suchman EA. Social Patterns of Illness and Medical Care. *J Health & Human Behavior* 6:2–16, 1965.
18. Kosa J, Antonovsky A, Zola I. *Poverty and Health.* (Cambridge: Harvard University Press, 1969).
19. Riessman F, Cohen J, Pearl M. *Mental Health of the Poor.* (New York: Free Press of Glencoe, 1964).
20. Deshaies J, Korper S, Siker E. Census Use Study. Report No. 12, *Health Information System II,* Bureau of the Census, US Dept of Commerce,
21. Zonana H, Henisz JE, Levine M. Psychiatric Emergency Service, A Decade Later. *Psychiatry in Medicine* 3:273–290, 1973.
22. Tischler GL, Henisz JE, Myers J, Garrison V. Catchmenting and Use of Mental Health Services. *Arch Gen Psychiat.* 27:389–392, 1972.
23. Tischler GL, Henisz JE, Myers J, Garrison V. The Impact of Catchmenting. *Administration in Mental Health* 1:22–29, 1972.
24. Tryon RC. *Identification of Social Areas by Cluster Analysis.* (Berkeley and Los Angeles: University of California Press, 1955).

25. Wolford JH, Hitchcock J, et al. The Effect on State Hospitalization of a Community Mental Health/Mental Retardation Center. *Amer J Psychiat.* 202–206, 1972.

Chapter five

1. Mechanic D: Response factors in illness: The study of illness behavior. *Soc Psychiat,* 1:11–20, 1966.
2. Suchman E: Social patterns of illness and medical care. *J Health Hum Behav,* 6:2–16, 1965.
3. Zola IK: Culture and symptoms: An analysis of patients' presenting complaints. *Amer Soc Rev,* 31:615–630, 1966.
4. Suchman EA: *Evaluative Research Principles and Practice in Public Service and Social Action Programs.* (New York: Russell Sage Foundation, 1967).
5. Donabedian A (ed): *Evaluating the Quality of Medical Care: A Guide to Medical Care Administration, Vol II.* (New York: APHA, 1970).
6. Garner EA, Miles HC, Iker HP, Romano J: A cumulative register of psychiatric services in a community. *AJPH* 53:1269–1277, 1963.
7. Donabedian A: Evaluating the quality of medical care. *Milb Mem Fund Quart,* 44:166–203, 1966.
8. Morehead MA: The medical audit as an operational tool. *AJPH,* 57:1643–1656, 1967.
9. Lembke PA: Medical auditing by scientific methods. *JAMA,* 162: 646–655, 1956.
10. Payne BC (ed): *Hospital Utilization Review Manual,* (Ann Arbor: University of Michigan Medical School, 1968).
11. Riedel DC, Brauer L, Brenner MH, Goldblatt P, Klerman G, Myers JK, Schwartz C: Developing a system for utilization review and evaluation in community mental health centers. *Hosp Comm Psychiat,* 22:229–232, 1971.
12. Zusman J, Slawson MR. The service quality profile. *Arch Gen Psychiatr,* 27:692–698, 1973.
13. Lee RI, Jones LW. *The Fundamentals of Good Medical Care.* (Chicago: University of Chicago Press, 1933).
14. Mikelbank G: Approval by individual diagnosis (AID) program, New Jersey Blue Cross. Paper presented at workshop in medical care — operational aspects. *APHA,* New York, Nov 11–12, 1966.
15. Babigian HM, Gardner EA, Miles HC, Romano J. Diagnostic consistency in a follow-up study of 1215 patients. *Amer J Psychiat,* 121:895–901, 1965.
16. Beck AT, Ward CH, Mendelson M, Mock J, Erbaugh J: Reliability of psychiatric diagnosis. *Amer J Psychiat,* 119:351–357, 1962.
17. Kendall RE, Cooper JE, Gourlay JRM, Copelan LS, Gurland BJ. Diagnostic criteria of American and British psychiatrists. *Arch Gen Psychiat,* 25:123–130, 1971.
18. Schmidt HO, Fonda CP: The reliability of psychiatric diagnosis: A new look. *J Abnorm Soc Psychol,* 52:262–267, 1956.

19. Silverman C. *The Epidemiology of Depression.* (Baltimore: The Johns Hopkins University Press, 1968).
20. Ward CH, Beck AT, Mendelson M, Mock JE, Erbaugh J. The psychiatric nomenclature: Reasons for diagnostic disagreement. *Arch Gen Psychiat,* 7:198–205, 1962.
21. Spitzer R, Endicott J. Diagno II: Further developments in a computer program for psychiatric diagnoses. *Amer J Psychiat,* 7 (Jan supp.) 12–21, 1969.
22. Lyerly SB, Abbot PS. *Handbook of Psychiatric Rating Scales (1959–1964).* Public Health Service Publication No. 1485. US Govt Printing Office, Washington, DC, 1966.
23. Astrachan BM, Harrow M, Adler D, Brauer L, Schwartz A, Schwartz C, Tucker G. A checklist for the diagnosis of schizophrenia. *Brit J Psychiat,* 121: 529–539, 1972.
24. Robbins E, Guze SD. Establishment of diagnostic validity in psychiatric illness: Its application to schizophrenia. *Amer J Psychiat,* 126: 983–987, 1970.
25. Feighner JP, Robins E, Guze SD, Woodruff RA, Winokur G, Munoz R. Diagnostic criteria for use in psychiatric research. *Arch Gen Psychiat,* 26:57–63, 1972.
26. Moss GR, Boren JJ. Specifying criteria for completion of psychiatric treatment. *Arch Gen Psychiat,* 24:441–447, 1971.
27. Hesbacher PT, Rickels K, Weise W. Target symptoms. *Arch Gen Psychiat,* 18:595–600, 1968.
28. Kiresuk TJ, Sherman RE. Goal attainment scaling: A general method for evaluating comprehensive community mental health programs. *Comm Ment Health J,* 4:443–453, 1968.
29. Community mental health data systems—A description of existing programs. *NIMH Mental Health Statistics.* Series C No. 2, Public Health Service publication No. 1990, 132–137, 1969.
30. Hogarty GW, Ulrich R. The discharge readiness inventory. *Arch Gen Psychiat,* 26: 419–426, 1972.

Chapter six

1. Goldblatt P, Brauer L, Garrison V, Henisz J, Malcolm-Lawes M. A Chart Review Checklist for Utilization Review in a Community Mental Health Center. *Hospital and Community Psychiatry* 24:753–756, 1973.
2. Richardson, F McD. Peer Review of Medical Care. *Medical Care* 10:29–39, 1972.
3. Henisz J, Goldblatt P, Flynn H, Garrison V. A Comparison of Three Approaches to Patient Care Appraisal Based on Chart Review. *Am J Psychiat.,* (in press).
4. Newman DE, Goldstein HS, Kazanjian V. A 1½ Year Experience with Peer Utilization Review. Read at the 126th Annual Meeting of the Amer Psychiatr Assn, Honolulu, 1973.

5. Meldmon MJ, Novick R, Squire M. Evaluation of the Psychiatrist's Performance. Read at the 126th Annual Meeting of the Amer Psychiatr Assn, Honolulu, 1973.

Chapter seven
1. Hardwick CP, Wolfe H: *A Psychiatric Utilization Review Program in Western Pennsylvania: An Evaluation of the Feasibility of Obtaining Data for Computerized Screening Models,* Final Report, HSM 110-70-314. (Pittsburgh: Blue Cross of Western Pennsylvania Research Department, 1972).
2. CUPIS, Connecticut Utilization and Patient Information Statistical System.
3. Riedel DC, Fetter RB, Mills RE, Pallett PJ: Basic Utilization Review Program (BURP), (New Haven: Health Services Research Program, Institution for Social and Policy Studies, Yale University), Working Paper 21, 1972.
4. Carlisle JH: AUTOGRP—A training program for the beginning AUTOGRP user. (New Haven: Health Services Research Program Institution for Social and Policy Studies, Yale University, 1973).
5. Mills RE, Fetter RB, Riedel DC, Brauer LO, Averill RF, Carlisle JH, Adler DA, Mills LM: AUTOGRP: An interactive system. (New Haven: Health Services Research Program, Institution for Social and Policy Studies, Yale University, 1973), Working Paper 23.
6. Astrachan BM, Adler DA, Brauer LO, Schwartz A, Schwartz CC, Tucker G. A checklist for the diagnosis of schizophrenia. *Brit J. Psychiat,* 121: 529-539, 1972.

Chapter eight
1. MacMahon, B. and Pugh, T.F. *Epidemiology: Principles and Methods.* (Boston: Little, Brown & Co., 1970), pp. 29-46.
2. Lilienfeld, A.M., Pedersen, E., Dowd, J.E. *Cancer Epidemiology: Methods of Study.* (Baltimore: The Johns Hopkins University Press, 1967), pp. 69-84.
3. Weissman, M.M., Paykel, E.S., French, N., Mark, H., Fox, K., and Prusoff, B. Suicide attempts in an urban community, 1955 and 1970. *Social Psychiatry* 8:82-91, 1973.
4. Rubenstein, R., Moses, R., and Lidz, T. On attempted suicide. *Arch. Gen. Psychiat.,* 79: 103-112, 1958.
5. Stengel, E. *Suicide and Attempted Suicide.* (Middlesex, England: Penguin Books, 1964).
6. Weissman, M.M. The epidemiology of suicide attempts, 1960-1971. *Arch. Gen. Psychiat.,* in press, 1974.
7. Fox, K. and Weissman, M. Suicide attempts and drugs: Contradiction between method and intent. Paper presented at the 50th Annual Meeting, American Orthopsychiatric Association, May 30, 1973, New York, N.Y.
8. Paykel, E.S., Hallowell, C., Dressler, D., Shapiro, D., and Weissman, M.M.

Treatment of suicide attempters: A descriptive study. Submitted for publication.

9. Bogard, M. Follow-up study of suicidal patients seen in emergency room consultation. *Amer. J. Psychiat.* 126: 1017–1020, 1970.

10. James, I.P., Derham, S.P., Scott-Orr, D.N. Attempted suicide—A study of 100 patients referred to a general hospital. *Med. J. Aust.* 1:375–380, 1963.

11. Stanley, W.J. Attempted suicide and suicidal gestures. *Brit. J. prev. soc. Med.* 23: 190–195, 1969.

12. Dressler, D.M., Prusoff, B.A., Mark, H., and Shapiro, D. Clinician attitudes towards the suicide attempter. Submitted for publication.

13. Weissman, M.M., Fox, K. and Klerman, G.L. Hostility and depression associated with suicide attempts. *Amer. J. Psychiat.* 130:450–455, 1973.

14. Tischler, G.L. and Riedel, D.C. A criterion oriented approach to patient care evaluation. *Amer. J. Psychiat.* 130:913–916, 1973.

15. Kirstein, L., Prusoff, B.A., Weissman, M.M., Dressler, D. Utilization review and suicide attempters: A comparison of explicit criteria and clinical practice. Amer. J. Psychiat. in press.

Chapter nine

1. Donabedian, A., "Evaluating the Quality of Medical Care," *Milbank Memorial Fund Quart.* 44 (pt. 2): 166–206, 1966.

2. Zusman, J. and Ross, E.R.R., "Evaluation of the Quality of Mental Health Services," *Arch Gen Psychiat,* 20: 353–357, 1969.

3. Deniston, O.L., Rosenstock, I.M., and Getting, V.A., "Evaluation of Program Effectiveness," *Public Health Reports,* 83:4, 323–335, 1968.

4. Riedel, D.C., Brauer, L., Brenner, M.H., Goldblatt, P., Schwartz, C., Myers, J.K., and Klerman, G., "Developing a System for Utilization Review and Evaluation in Community Mental Health Centers," *Hospital and Community Psychiatry,* 22:8, 229–232, 1971.

5. Schwartz, C.C., Myers, J.K., and Astrachan, B.M., "The Outcome Study in Psychiatric Evaluation Research: Issues and Method," *Arch. Gen. Psychiat.* 29:98–105, 1973.

6. May, P.R.A., Tuma, A.H., and Kraude, W., "Community Follow-Up of Treatment of Schizophrenia—Issues and Problems," *Amer. J. Orthopsychiat,* 35:754–763, 1965.

7. May, P.R.A., *Treatment of Schizophrenia.* (New York: Science House, 1968).

8. Sandifer, M.G., Hordern, A., Tinbury, G.C., and Green, L.M., "Psychiatric Diagnosis: A Comparative Study in North Carolina, London, and Glasgow," *Brit J. Psychiat,* 114:1–9, 1968.

9. Astrachan, B.M., Harrow, M., Adler, D., Brauer, L., Schwartz, A., Schwartz, C., and Tucker, G., "A Checklist for the Diagnosis of Schizophrenia," *Brit J. Psychiat,* 121: 529–539, 1972.

10. Spitzer, R.L. and Endicott, J., "Diagno II: Further Developments in a Computer Program for Psychiatric Diagnosis," *Amer J. Psychiat,* 125:7, 12–21, 1969.

11. Paykel, E.S., Klerman, G.L., and Prusoff, B.A., "Treatment Setting and Clinical Depression," *Arch Gen Psychiat*, 22: 11–21, 1970.

12. Vaillant, G.E., "The Prediction of Recovery in Schizophrenia," *J Nerv Ment Dis*, 135: 534–543, 1962.

13. Vaillant, G.E., "Prospective Prediction of Schizophrenic Remission," *Arch Gen Psychiat*, 22: 509–518, 1964.

14. Stephens, J.H. and Astrup, C., "Prognosis in 'Process' and 'Non-Process' Schizophrenia," *Amer J Psychiat*, 119: 945–952, 1963.

15. Myers, J.K., Lindenthal, J.J., and Pepper, M.P., "Life Events and Psychiatric Impairment," *J. Nerv Ment Dis*, 152: 149–157, 1971.

16. Bock, R.D., "Multivariate Analysis of Variance of Repeated Measurements," in C.W. Harris (ed.) *Problems in Measuring Change*. (Madison: University of Wisconsin Press, 1963).

17. Armor, D.J. and Couch, A.S., *The Data-Text Primer: An Introduction to Computerized Social Data Analysis Using the Data-Text System*. (New York: The Free Press, 1972.)

18. Group for the Advancement of Psychiatry, "Some Observations on Controls in Psychiatric Research," Report #42, 1959.

19. Hyman, H., *Survey Design and Analysis*. (New York: The Free Press, 1955.)

20. Myers, J.K., Schwartz, C.C., Brauer, L., Brenner, M.H., "The Outcome of Schizophrenia: A Follow-Up Study," in preparation.

21. Hollingshead, A.B. and Redlich, F.C., *Social Class and Mental Illness*. (New York: John Wiley and Sons, 1958).

22. Klerman, G.L., and Paykel, E.S., "Depressive Pattern, Social Background and Hospitalization," *J Nerv Ment Dis*, 150: 466–478, 1970.

23. Schwartz, C.C., Brenner, M.H., and Myers, J.K., "Social Adjustment and the Outcome of Schizophrenia," in preparation.

24. O'Brien, C.P., Hamm, K.B., Ray, B.A., Pierce, J.F., Luborsky, L., Mintz, J., "Group vs. Individual Psychotherapy with Schizophrenics," *Arch Gen Psychiat*, 27: 474–478, 1972.

25. May, P.R.A., and Tuma, A.H., "Choice of Criteria for the Assessment of Treatment Outcome," *J. Psychiat. Res.*, 2:199–209, 1964.

26. Prusoff, B.A., Klerman, G.L., Paykel, E.S., "Concordance Between Clinical Assessments and Patients' Self Report in Depression," *Arch. Gen. Psychiat.*, 26: 546–552, 1972.

27. Keniston, K., Boltax, S., Almond, R., "Multiple Criteria of Treatment Outcome," *J. Psychiat. Res.*, 8:107–118, 1971.

28. Ellsworth, R.B., and Clayton, W.H., "Measurement of Improvement in Mental Illness," *J. Consult. Psychol.*, 23: 15–20, 1959.

29. Schooler, N.R., Goldberg, S.C., Boothe, H., Cole, J.O., "One Year after Discharge: Community Adjustment of Schizophrenic Patients," *Amer. J. Psychiat.*, 123:986–995, February 1967.

30. Strauss, J.S. and Carpenter, W.T., "The Prediction of Outcome in Schizophrenia," *Arch. Gen. Psychiat.* 27: 739–746, 1972.

31. Myers, J.K. Lidenthal, J.J. and Pepper, M.P., "Life Events and Psychiatric Impairment," *J. Nerv. Ment. Dis.*, 152: 149–157, 1971.

32. Srole, L., Langner, T.S., Michael, S.T., Opler, M.K., and Rennie, T.A.C., *Mental Health in the Metropolis: The Midtown Manhattan Study,* vol. 1. (New York: McGraw Hill, 1962).
33. Leighton, D.C., Harding, J.S., Macklin, D.B., Macmillan, A.M. and Leighton, A.H., *The Character of Danger: The Stirling County Study of Psychiatric Disorder and Sociocultural Environment, III.* (New York: Basic Books, 1963).
34. Dohrenwend, B., *Social Status and Psychological Disorder: A Causal Inquiry.* (New York: John Wiley and Sons, 1969).
35. Kubie, L., "The Fundamental Nature of the Distinction Between Normality and Neurosis," *Psych. Quart.,* 23: 167–203, quote, 182–183, 1954.
36. Hartmann, H., "Psycho-Analysis and the Concept of Health," *Int. J. of Psycho.,* 20: 308–321, 1939.
37. Erikson, E., "Growth and Crises of the Healthy Personality," in Kluckhohn, Murray, and Schneider, (eds.) *Personality in Nature Society, and Culture,* (New York: Alfred A. Knopf, 1964).
38. Zubin, J., "Evaluation of Therapeutic Outcome in Mental Disorders," *J. Nerv. Ment. Dis.,* 117: 95–111, 1953.
39. Parsons, T., "Definitions of Health and Illness in the Light of American Values and Social Structure," in *Social Structure and Personality.* (New York: The Free Press of Glencoe, 1964) pp. 257–291.
40. Gurin, G., Veroff, J., Feld, S., *American View Their Mental Health.* (New York: Basic Books, 1960).
41. Endicott, J., Spitzer, R.L., "What! Another Rating Scale? The Psychiatric Evaluation Form," *Journal of Nervous and Mental Disease,* 1972.
42. Schwartz, C.C., Myers, J.K., Astrachan, B.M., "Comparing Three Measures of Mental Status: A Note on the Validity of Estimates of Psychological Disorder in the Community,"*J. Health. Soc. Behav.,* 14: 265–273,1973.
43. Schwartz, C.C., Myers, J.K., Astrachan, B.M., "Concordance of Multiple Assessments of the Outcome of Schizophrenia," Arch. Gen. Psychiat. in press, 1974.

Chapter ten
1. Bank, R. The Multistate Information System: A tool for program monitoring. Paper presented at the Eighty-first Annual Convention of the American Psychological Association, Montreal, Canada, August 27–31, 1973.
2. Cytrynbaum, S. The review and evaluation of consultation activities in a community mental health center: Pitfalls and possibilities. Unpublished paper, Department of Psychiatry, Yale University, 1974.
3. Information Sciences Division, Rockland State Hospital, *Multistate Information System For Psychiatric Patients.* (New York: Research Foundation for Mental Hygiene, 1973).
4. Jaques, E. Social systems as defense against persecutory and depressive anxiety. In M. Klein (ed.) *New Directions in Psychoanalysis.* (New York: Basic Books, 1955).

5. Menzies, I. A case study in the functioning of social systems as a defense against anxiety. *Human Relations, 13,* 1960, 95–121.

6. Miller, E.J. and Rice, A.K. *Systems of Organizations;* (London: Tavistock Publications, 1967).

7. National Institutes of Mental Health. *Definition of Terms in Mental Health, Alcohol Abuse, Drug Abuse and Mental Retardation: Mental Health Statistics Series No. 8.* (Rockville, Maryland: U.S. Department of Health, Education and Welfare, 1973).

8. Nelson, R.H. and Burgess, T.H. An open adaptive systems analysis of community mental health services. *Social Psychiatry,* in press.

9. Newton, P.M. and Levinson, D.T. The work group within the organization: A sociopsychological approach. *Psychiatry, 36:* 115–142, 1973.

10. Norman, E.C. and Forti, T.J. A study of the process and the outcome of mental health consultation. *Community Mental Health Journal 8* (4): 261–270, 1972.

11. Rice, A.K. Individual, group and intergroup processes, *Human Relations, 22:* 565–584, 1969.

Index

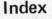

About the Editors

Donald C. Riedel, Ph.D., is Professor of Public Health (Medical Care) in the School of Medicine and the Institution for Social and Policy Studies, Yale University. He completed his graduate work in Sociology at Purdue University and has, for more than fifteen years, been conducting research, teaching, and consulting in the area of patient care and program evaluation in various institutional and ambulatory settings. He is the author or co-author of numerous publications in the field.

Jerome K. Myers, Professor of Sociology at Yale University, has been a member of an interdisciplinary research team of sociologists and psychiatrists at Yale studying relationships between social class and mental illness since 1950. He is presently Director of Graduate Studies in Sociology at Yale. He is a consultant to a variety of health organizations and past Chairman of the Medical Sociology section of the American Sociological Association.

Dr. Myers received his B.A. (1942) in Sociology from Franklin and Marshall College in Lancaster, Pa., and both his M.A. (1947) and Ph.D. (1950) from Yale.

Dr. Myers is the co-author of A DECADE LATER, FAMILY AND CLASS DYNAMICS IN MENTAL ILLNESS and AN EMPIRICAL APPROACH TO THE STUDY OF SCHIZOPHRENIA and the author of numerous book chapters and journal articles.

Gary L. Tischler, M.D., is at present Associate Professor of Clinical Psychiatry in the Department of Psychiatry, Yale University School of Medicine; Director of the Department's Social and Community Psychiatry Program and Associate Director of The Connecticut Mental Health Center.

A graduate of the University of Pennsylvania Medical School, Dr. Tischler's psychiatric residency was at Yale University. He joined the faculty in 1967 and was majorally involved in the planning and development of a federally funded community mental health program, the Hill-West Haven Division.

His research interests lie in the area of program evaluation and he has written extensively on the issues concerning the interface between program and community, psychiatric utilization review, and the evaluation of mental health services.